GLUTEN-FREE MEAL PREP COOKBOOK

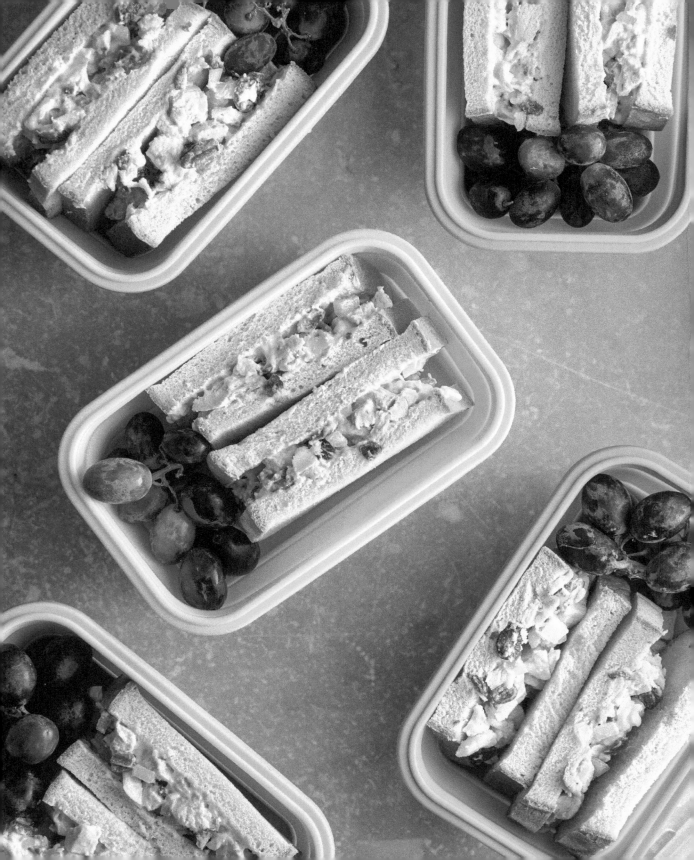

GLUTEN-FREE
MEAL PREP
—≡— COOKBOOK —≡—

Time-Saving Plans and
Easy, Affordable Recipes

Pam Wattenbarger

PHOTOGRAPHY BY DARREN MUIR

ROCKRIDGE
PRESS

For general information on our other products and services or to obtain technical support, please contact our Customer Care Department within the United States at (866) 744-2665, or outside the United States at (510) 253-0500.

Rockridge Press publishes its books in a variety of electronic and print formats. Some content that appears in print may not be available in electronic books, and vice versa.

Interior and Cover Designer: Stephanie Mautone
Art Producer: Janice Ackerman
Editor: Myryah Irby
Production Editor: Ashley Polikoff
Photography: © 2020 Darren Muir. Food styling by Yolanda Muir.

ISBN: Print 978-1-64739-980-1 | eBook 978-1-64739-981-8
R0

To Bryan, Brittany, Justin, Ashton, and Critter—
the reasons I learned allergy-friendly cooking techniques

Contents

PART 2

Prep Yourself: Preparing Customized Meal Preps 149

Rise and Shine: Breaking for Breakfast 151

Take Time to Nourish: Lunch and Dinner 161

Recipes to Relish: Sauces, Dressings, and Dips 177

Nibbles and Noshes: Snacks and Desserts 187

Introduction

Cooking nutritious meals on a daily basis can be a challenge. Add food allergies to the mix or the need for a gluten-free diet, and it becomes even harder. Sometimes in the midst of a hectic schedule, it's easier to order delivery or takeout, but the cost of those meals can add up quickly—both to your wallet and to your health.

I'm Pam Wattenbarger, and I began my gluten-free cooking journey in 2011 when my daughter was diagnosed with celiac disease. At the time, few gluten-free options were available in stores. Almost everything I prepared had to be made from scratch. With many of my family's traditional meals off the table—literally—I had to find recipes the entire family would enjoy. That meant spending a lot of time in the kitchen experimenting with traditional recipes and creating new ones. The only problem? I didn't have hours to spend in the kitchen.

One day, while making a spaghetti pie and a spare to keep in the freezer for emergencies, a light bulb went off. "Why not make five days' meals at once?" I tried my plan, spending four or five hours one Saturday afternoon preparing main dishes. The next week, dinnertime was a breeze. I'd pull out a container of something like my Spicy Salsa Chili (page 163) and put it on the stove to simmer while I baked a pan of corn bread.

My family appreciates my meal prep efforts, too, especially as their list of food allergies continues to expand. They're able to request favorite dishes during our weekly preps. We're also able to expand our repertoire with new recipes on a regular basis. When I'm out of town working as a travel writer, meals prepped in advance mean my family won't eat out *every* night while I'm away.

I'm not the only one that's sold on meal prep. It's seen a rise in popularity as more people try to create healthy, cost-effective, allergy-friendly meals at home. However, beginning a meal prep plan can be daunting. Where do you start? What should you prep and in which order? What types of dishes can you prep, and how do you store them?

You'll learn the answers to these questions and more here. From the first step of deciding which day to shop and cook to the last step of storing food,

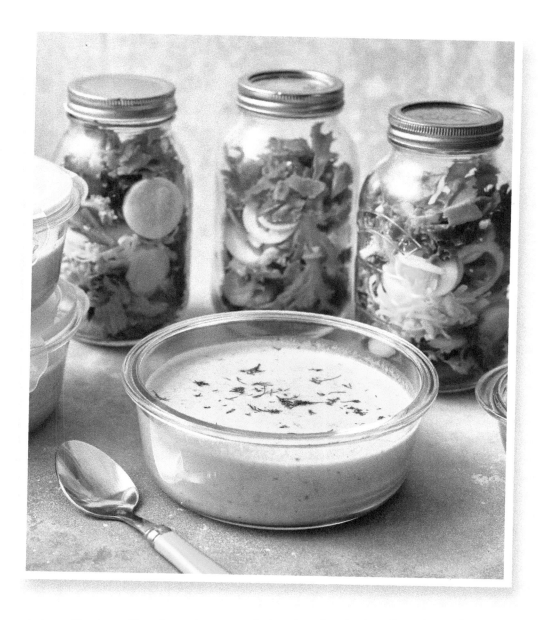

I share the benefits of meal prep and step-by-step instructions to walk you through every aspect of the process. Soon, you'll be able to use these steps to branch out and develop your own meal prep plans.

Whether you're new to meal prepping or a seasoned pro, this book will give you the tools to start eating healthier meals, spending less money on them, and enjoying more time outside the kitchen.

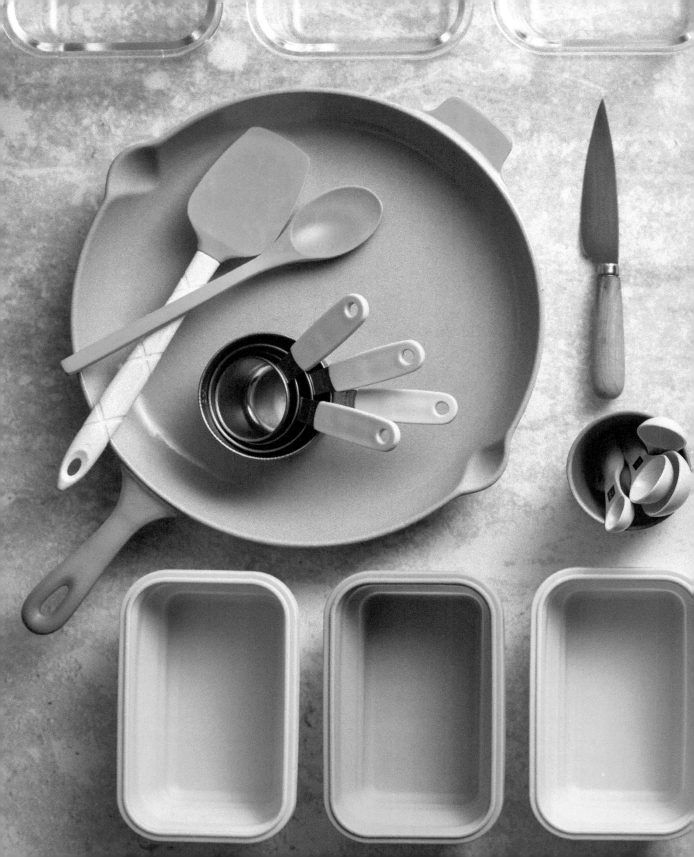

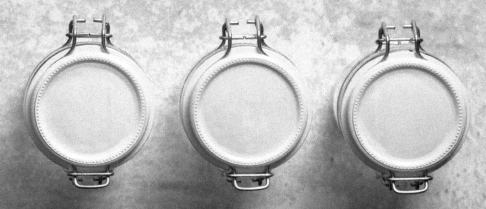

PART 1

Gluten-Free
Made Easy

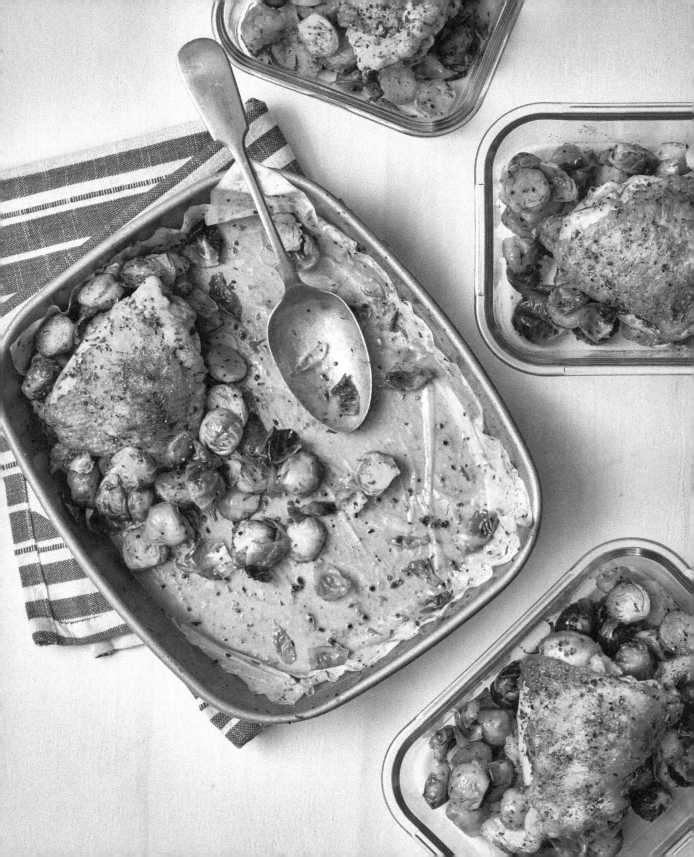

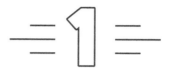

Prepping for Success

Are you tired of debating what to cook each night? Would you like to spend less time in the kitchen? Do your meals lack variety? You're not alone. Maybe you've tried a menu plan—planning daily menus of different meals for a week or a month at a time—and it didn't work. Meal prep is different. It involves spending a concentrated amount of time cooking meals one day a week and, if you feel like it, portioning the meals into individual servings to consume throughout the week.

‹‹ Herbed Sheet Pan Chicken with Brussels Sprouts, page 77

Meal Prep 101

At first, spending several hours in the kitchen might seem like a chore, but it's worth the time investment. Once you've finished the prep, you'll have four or five days of breakfasts, lunches, and dinners, including garnishes, toppings, and condiments, at your fingertips, safely stored in the refrigerator or freezer. Imagine what you'll do with all the time you've just freed up during the week.

Ready to begin your meal prep journey? This chapter provides the tips you need to succeed.

What Does It Mean to Be Gluten-Free?

A gluten-free diet eliminates gluten—a protein found in wheat, rye, barley, triticale, and sometimes oats, depending on how it's processed. People eliminate gluten from their diet for a variety of reasons. For some people with celiac disease or gluten sensitivities, a small amount of gluten in food is enough to cause significant health issues. Others eliminate gluten to promote weight loss or boost their energy.

Although there are more gluten-free products on the market today than ever before, some of them, including teff flour or amaranth flour, are not readily available at many local stores. To use these flours in recipes, several varieties must be mixed together, creating an expensive blend. Other groceries may have a handful of products with little variety.

When I began to prepare gluten-free meals, I learned to read labels. Because gluten is a binding agent and helps foods maintain their shape, many packaged foods contain gluten. It often shows up in unexpected places, like dressing mixes or soups. Other foods are made on production lines that may have come in contact with wheat or other gluten-containing foods, meaning cross-contamination can be a problem.

This meant I had to choose items that were naturally gluten-free, such as meat, produce, and vegetables. If my family wanted "traditional" dishes, I had to plan, experiment with recipes, and keep supplies on hand. Meal prep became an essential part of my gluten-free cooking process.

Over time, I realized we were eating fewer processed meals, saving money thanks to less-frequent grocery shopping, and trying new recipes. Both our health and our wallet were thankful.

Feeling Preppy: Meal Prep Benefits

Reducing the daily stress of meal planning is only one of the benefits of meal prep.

- **You'll eat healthier and avoid gluten.** Meal prep helps you be intentional about what—and how much—you're eating. By planning and portioning ahead, you can pack individual servings and set yourself up for a successful week. For those with gluten sensitivities or other food allergies, meal prepping ensures all of your meals are gluten-free and allergy friendly.

- **You can maximize your time.** Planning to cook and shop on one day helps streamline the time you'll spend at the store each week. You'll also save time in the kitchen on a daily basis.

- **You will save money.** According to a study by the United States Department of Agriculture, Americans spend almost 10 percent of their disposable income on food. Often, we don't realize how much money we spend at the grocery store when purchasing a few items several times a week or buying an impulse fast-food meal. Using an itemized shopping list prevents you from wandering the aisles deciding what to cook or reaching for expensive packaged convenience foods in a pinch.

- **You will begin to eliminate food waste.** A 2020 study by Pennsylvania State University reported that the average American wastes 30 to 40 percent of the food they purchase. And the cost of that food waste—tossing leftovers or forgetting food in the refrigerator until it goes bad—adds up quickly. Meal prep helps eliminate this by ensuring you'll be purchasing only the amount of food you'll need and reusing the same ingredients across several meals.

- **You will add variety to your diet.** By planning meals, you can look for new recipes or new ingredients you'd like to try. Rotate through the seasonal meal-prep recipes in this book, and you'll have several weeks of no-repeat meals. Add your favorite recipes to the meal plan when you feel comfortable with the prep.

The recipes and meal prep plans in this book are designed to take a few hours to complete after shopping for the ingredients. The four-recipe plans should take about 2 hours, the five-recipe plans should take about 2½ hours, and the six-recipe plans should take about 3 hours. At first, the recipes might take a little longer than the allotted time to prepare. Once you get the hang of prepping, however, you'll become more efficient at multitasking, resulting in less time spent in the kitchen.

Packaging and Storing

Instructions on how to pack and store the meals are included at the end of each recipe. You can choose to pack the recipe into individual servings or into one container that serves four, whichever is best for you. If you want or need more servings of a particular dish, double or triple the recipe.

For meal prep to work successfully, proper containers are needed to store your food. I share detailed tips about containers and storage on pages 6 and 7. Containers don't have to be expensive. There's a selection for every budget. Begin with a few containers, and expand your collection over time. If your family, like mine, tends to "misplace" containers and lids, choose budget-friendly brands. If you can never find the right lid for the container you want to use, invest in containers with attached lids. Another option is to purchase a small set of containers in different sizes and expand your collection as you find the containers that best fit your needs.

Stock Up and Save: The Gluten-Free Pantry

Have you ever decided to prepare a recipe, gone to your pantry, and discovered you are missing a key ingredient? When that happens, it's all too easy to abandon your plan rather than make a trip to the grocery store. Stocking the pantry not only makes meal prep easier but also saves money. Who hasn't dashed into a store for "one or two items" and returned with a full bag?

Here is a list of staple ingredients to keep on hand to prepare recipes in this book. As your meal-prep repertoire expands to include your favorite dishes, add more ingredients for variety.

- All-purpose gluten-free one-to-one baking flour

- Baking powder

- Baking soda

- Canned vegetables, including:

  - ☐ *Beans: black beans, chili, green, and kidney*

  - ☐ *Seasoned diced tomatoes*

  - ☐ *Tomato sauce*

  - ☐ *Whole kernel corn*

- Cornstarch

- Dried herbs, spices, and extracts: Purchase the basics listed here, and add to your collection over time.

  - ☐ *Black pepper: purchase peppercorns with a built-in grinder for freshly ground*

  - ☐ *Curry powder*

  - ☐ *Dried basil*

  - ☐ *Dried parsley*

  - ☐ *Dried thyme*

  - ☐ *Garlic powder*

  - ☐ *Ground cinnamon*

  - ☐ *Italian seasoning*

- ☐ *Onion powder*

- ☐ *Paprika*

- ☐ *Red pepper flakes*

- ☐ *Sea salt*

- ☐ *Vanilla extract*

- Gluten-free pasta

- Lentils, brown or green

- Oil: extra-virgin olive oil and canola oil

- Peanut butter, or other nut or seed butter of choice

- Quinoa

- Rice, long-grain white and basmati

- Salsa

- Sweeteners: brown and granulated sugars; liquid sweetener such as agave, honey, or molasses

- Unsweetened cocoa powder

- Nonstick cooking spray

- Vinegar: balsamic, distilled white

Always check ingredient packaging for gluten-free labeling (in order to ensure foods, especially oats, were processed in a completely gluten-free facility).

Sensible Storage

Successful meal prep needs proper storage space for your food and proper containers in which to store the food. Although you do have to invest in storage, it doesn't have to be a costly up-front expenditure. Start small. Begin in your kitchen. Take an inventory to assess the containers you have: How many? What sizes? Matching lids? Purchase additional containers as needed.

Another important element in meal prep is labeling. No one wants to find a UFO (unidentified freezer object). Fancy labels aren't necessary—unless that's what you want. You can use a Sharpie, dry-erase marker, or chalk pens to achieve the same results. Or, if you prefer, create reusable labels using a label maker. And—here's a trick I learned from a chef—use rubbing alcohol to remove the writing from the lid before washing the container.

Containers

Important attributes: No matter which type of containers you choose, be sure they are leakproof and microwave/freezer/dishwasher friendly. A leakproof container helps avoid food waste and prevents nasty spills. Microwave-friendly containers mean you have easy reheating options, and dishwasher-friendly containers mean cleanup is a breeze.

Number of containers: Start with at least five containers, and add more based on how the meals are prepped. Do you plan to portion the meals into individual servings? Into meals for a family of four? Perhaps you plan a mix of both. Use these general guidelines to determine the number of containers you need.

- 5 dinners packaged for a family of four: 5 large (32-ounce) containers

- 5 dinners packaged in individual servings: 20 (8-ounce) containers

- 5 dinners packaged in a mixture of individual and family servings: 2 large (32-ounce) containers and 12 individual (8-ounce) containers

- 4 small (1- to 2-ounce) containers to hold dressings and toppings

TYPES OF CONTAINERS

- **Glass:** Options range from traditional glass storage bowls to Mason jars in 4-, 8-, 16-, or 32-ounce sizes. Mason jars are a good choice for layered salads and smoothies. Mini (1-ounce) Mason jars are good for dressings. If you use glass bowls with lids, remember they are not designed to withstand high heat or sudden changes in temperature. Heating the bowl directly from the freezer could cause breakage.

MUST-HAVE KITCHEN TOOLS

Whether you're a novice or a seasoned cook, these kitchen essentials will provide almost every tool you need to prepare delicious and healthy meals.

- **Baking dishes:** 9-by-9-inch, 9-by-13-inch

- **Blender**

- **Bowls:**

    - ☐ *Microwave-safe: small, medium, and large*

    - ☐ *Mixing: small, medium, and large*

- **Cutting board:** Wood lasts longer, but plastic costs less up front.

- **Knives:** chef's knife, paring knife, and serrated knife

- **Measuring cups:** I like to have two of these—one for wet ingredients and one for dry ingredients. The glass measuring cups work well for wet ingredients, and the individual stainless steel or plastic cups, usually available in ¼-, ⅓-, ½-, and 1-cup sizes, work well for dry ingredients.

- **Measuring spoons:** either stainless steel or plastic, usually in a set of five, including ⅛, ¼, ½, and 1 teaspoon and 1 tablespoon

- **Mixer:** stand or handheld

- **Mixing spoons:** large wooden or silicone spoons

- **Pots and pans:** 2-quart and 4-quart saucepans, preferably with lids, stockpot or Dutch oven

- **Sheet pan**

- **Skillet:** 10-inch nonstick, preferably with a lid

- **Spatula:** I prefer silicone since it doesn't scratch nonstick pans, but metal spatulas work well on cast-iron skillets and withstand high temperatures without melting.

- **Nestable/stackable:** Nestable containers save valuable storage space when not in use, whereas stackable containers save space in the freezer.

- **Plastic:** Choose BPA-free reusable containers. In my kitchen, I use stackable rectangular containers with clear lids. They use less space in my freezer, can be microwaved or put in the dishwasher, and make the contents easy to see. A budget-friendly choice for family meal storage is Mainstays 15-piece meal prep containers. They're available in family-meal size (4 servings), in "deep dish" size for soups or salads, and with divided compartments. I use Ziploc Twist 'n Loc containers in various sizes for individual portions, toppings, and condiments.

- **Single- and multi-compartment:** Single-compartment containers are good for packaging family meals or, in smaller sizes, individual servings. Multiple-compartment containers hold both a main dish and a side for a complete meal.

Labeling

Label containers with the name of the dish. If you're preparing meals for people with special dietary needs, using notations such as gluten-free, dairy-free, peanut-free, shellfish-/fish-free, vegan, or vegetarian ensures everyone receives the correct meal. It's also important to add the date to the container lid before storing. This practice lets you know when food expires and helps prevent waste.

Thawing and Reheating

Once food has been packaged, it should only be stored for as long as indicated in the recipes or according to general guidelines if you're not following a particular recipe in this book. Most cooked foods have a freezer life of 1 to 3 months before showing signs of freezer burn, according to the Food and Drug Administration.

It's also important to know how to properly thaw and reheat food to prevent bacteria growth.

Casseroles, meats, seafood, dairy, and other perishable dishes should be thawed in the refrigerator. Put casseroles in the refrigerator 1 to 2 days in advance. Plan for 8 hours of thawing time per pound of meat, 6 hours per pound of fruits and vegetables, and 4 to 5 hours per pound of poultry.

- To reheat thawed casseroles in the microwave, loosely cover the microwave-safe dish with wax paper. Using the reheat button, heat for 3 minutes. Stir. If mixture has not warmed, heat for 1 more minute. The internal temperature should be 165°F.

- To thaw soups, stews, chilis, and other liquid dishes quickly, place the sealed container in a sink full of hot water until the food begins to separate from the sides.

- Baked goods, such as muffins, can be thawed at room temperature.

What Not to Prep

Not everything lends itself to food storage. Potatoes and gluten-free pasta tend to become "mushy" when reheated. The meals in this book are designed to keep and reheat well. In the recipes, we'll undercook the pasta and potatoes before storing so they finish cooking during the reheating process, or we'll store them separately.

Some fruits, such as apples, pears, bananas, and avocados, turn brown and, although safe to eat, look unappetizing. We'll use these ingredients in smoothies and baked dishes. Or in the case of the avocado, we'll prep a fresh one the day of eating instead of in advance.

How to Store Food Properly

It's important to prepare and store food properly to prevent bacteria and mold growth. Food poisoning is no fun! Thankfully, there are ways to prevent it. Warm foods should never go directly into the freezer because doing so can cause the surrounding items to partially thaw and refreeze. Instead, put the food in shallow, uncovered containers in the refrigerator. Once the food has cooled, remove it from the refrigerator, package it in airtight containers, and freeze it if you won't be consuming it within 3 to 5 days. It's best to place containers in a single layer in the freezer to allow air circulation and rapid freezing and avoid overcrowding.

FOOD	REFRIGERATOR	FREEZER
Bacon	7 days	1 month
Butter	3 months	6 months
Cheese, hard (Parmesan), unopened	6 months	6 months
Cheese, semi-hard (Cheddar, Havarti, Swiss), unopened	6 months	6 months
Cooked chicken: baked, barbecued, roasted	3 to 5 days	4 months
Cooked chicken dishes (casseroles)	3 to 5 days	4 months
Cooked meats and meat dishes	3 to 5 days	2 to 3 months
Egg frittata, omelets, quiche	3 to 5 days	2 months
Eggs, in the shell	3 to 5 weeks	Do not freeze
Eggs, raw yolks and whites	2 to 4 days	1 year
Fish, cooked	3 to 4 days	3 months
Fish, fatty	1 to 2 days	3 to 4 months
Fish, lean	1 to 2 days	6 to 8 months
Flours, almond, coconut	6 months	1 year
Fresh crab, scallops, shrimp, squid	1 to 2 days	3 to 6 months
Frozen fruit	N/A	8 to 12 months
Frozen vegetables	N/A	8 to 12 months
Ground meats: beef, chicken, lamb, pork, turkey	1 to 2 days	3 to 4 months
Meat: beef, lamb, pork	3 to 5 days	4 to 12 months
Milk	1 week	1 month
Nondairy milk	7 to 10 days	Do not freeze
Poultry (parts)	1 to 2 days	9 months
Sausage: beef, chicken, pork, turkey	1 to 2 days	1 to 2 months
Soups and stews, with meat	3 to 5 days	2 to 3 months
Soups and stews, vegetarian	3 to 5 days	3 months
Tofu, unopened	3 weeks	3 months
Yogurt, unopened	2 weeks	2 months

If you prefer, cool dishes slightly on the counter for 10 to 20 minutes before placing in the refrigerator. The maximum time perishable foods, such as meats, seafood, dairy, eggs, and most casseroles, can stay at room temperature is around 2 hours. If the temperature is above 90°F, the time at room temperature reduces to 1 hour. Baked goods, such as breads, muffins, and cookies, can typically be stored in airtight containers at room temperature for up to 4 days before going stale.

Prepping and Planning: About the Meal Prep Plans

When you're ready to begin, you'll find the book organized according to three types of meal plans:

☐ *Chapter 2 has four seasonal meal prep plans—one each for summer, spring, fall, and winter. These plans include four recipes and take about 2 hours to prep.*

☐ *Chapter 3 has four seasonal meal prep plans that include five recipes and take about 2½ hours to prep.*

☐ *Chapter 4 has four seasonal meal prep plans that include six recipes and take about 3 hours to prep.*

• Every meal plan will focus on interchangeable lunches and dinners and include breakfast. The meal plans in chapter 4 also include one snack or dessert. Seasonal produce is featured, but fresh produce can be replaced with canned or frozen, if needed.

• Each recipe includes dietary labels on the recipe page. Review the recipes before shopping to be sure they meet your dietary specifications and won't need ingredient swaps. Whenever possible, I add substitutions or tips.

- If you are new to meal prepping, begin with chapter 2, with the four-recipe meal prep plans. As you become more comfortable, work your way up to prepping more recipes.

- Although you can absolutely do these preps over and over, at some point you will crave variety. That's why I've also included extra recipes in part 2. They can be swapped into existing preps, added onto existing preps, or used to create custom preps.

Grab a pan and let's get cooking!

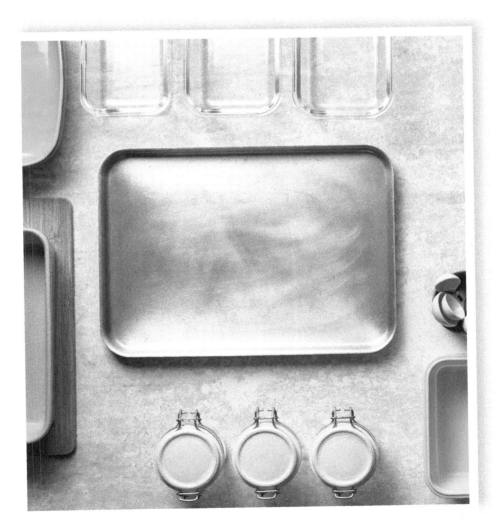

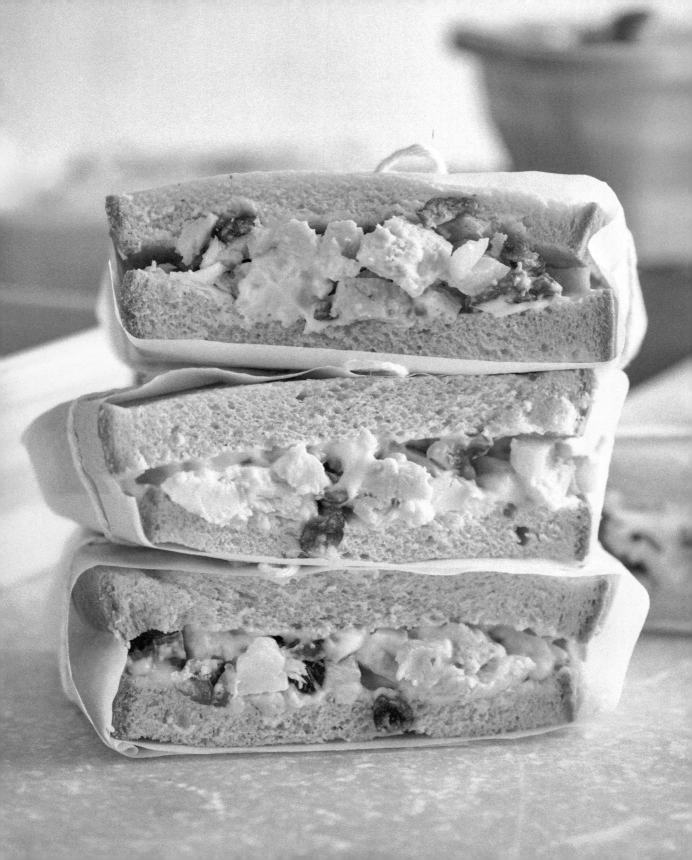

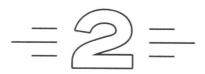

The Fabulous Four: Four-Recipe Meal Preps

Your first week of meal prep will give you a good idea of what to expect for the next three preps. We are going to start with a simple, tasty menu that's easy to adapt for food allergies and dietary preferences. Remember to shop your pantry and refrigerator first for items you have on hand, such as rice, garlic, spices, olive oil, and all-purpose gluten-free one-to-one baking flour. You can also substitute items, such as your favorite type of shredded cheese for the Cheddar cheese in this menu or sausage for bacon. Browse The Gluten-Free Pantry (page 4) before you begin and, if possible, purchase some of the staples you'll need. This will ensure you have basic supplies on hand to make the meal prep process easier. Our goal is to prepare meals that help you spend less time in the kitchen without sacrificing flavor.

‹‹ Cranberry and Pecan Chicken Salad, page 21

SPRING MENU:
Four-Recipe Meal Prep Shopping List

PRODUCE
Celery (1 bunch)
Garlic (1 head)
Mushrooms, cremini (1 [8-ounce] carton)
Onions, yellow (2)

DAIRY AND EGGS
Butter, salted (8 ounces)
Buttermilk, low-fat (1 pint)
Cheese, cottage, full-fat (1 [15-ounce] container)
Cheese, goat (1 [3-ounce] package)
Cheese, Cheddar, mild, shredded (1 [8-ounce] bag)
Eggs, large (1 half dozen)

MEAT
Bacon (1 [12-ounce] package)
Chicken, breasts, boneless, skinless (1 pound)

FROZEN FOOD
Broccoli (1 [10-ounce] package)
Shrimp, medium, peeled, deveined, tails off (1 pound)

CANNED AND BOTTLED
Broth, chicken (1 [32-ounce] container)
Maple syrup (1 [8-ounce] bottle)
Mayonnaise, full-fat (1 [5½-ounce] container)

PANTRY
Bread, gluten-free (1 loaf)
Cranberries, dried (1 cup)
Flour, all-purpose gluten-free one-to-one baking (1 [1-pound] package)
Pecans, raw, chopped (1 cup)
Rice, long-grain, white (1 [12-ounce] package)

CHECK YOUR PANTRY FOR . . .
Baking soda, black peppercorns, dried chives, extra-virgin olive oil, garlic powder, Italian seasoning, non-stick cooking spray, sea salt

Weekly Meal Chart

	BREAKFAST	LUNCH	DINNER
DAY 1	Savory Bacon and Cheddar Pancakes	Cranberry and Pecan Chicken Salad	Crustless Broccoli Quiche
DAY 2	Savory Bacon and Cheddar Pancakes	Shrimp and Mushroom Pilaf	Cranberry and Pecan Chicken Salad
DAY 3	Crustless Broccoli Quiche	Cranberry and Pecan Chicken Salad	Shrimp and Mushroom Pilaf
DAY 4	Savory Bacon and Cheddar Pancakes	Cranberry and Pecan Chicken Salad	Crustless Broccoli Quiche
DAY 5	Savory Bacon and Cheddar Pancakes	Shrimp and Mushroom Pilaf	Crustless Broccoli Quiche

STEP-BY-STEP PREP

1. Cook the chicken. In a large saucepan, combine 1 pound boneless, skinless chicken breasts and 3 cups chicken broth, or enough to completely cover the chicken, and bring to a boil over medium heat. Cook for 15 minutes, depending on the thickness of your chicken, or until it reaches an internal temperature of 165°F. Remove from the heat. Let cool for 5 minutes. Remove the chicken from the saucepan. Save the broth used to cook the chicken to use in soups and stews. It can be frozen in an airtight container for up to 6 months. Dice the chicken.

2. Cook the rice. Rinse the saucepan and return to medium heat. Combine 1⅓ cups water, ⅔ cup chicken broth, 1 cup long-grain white rice, 1 teaspoon sea salt, and ⅔ tablespoon butter. Cook for 7 to 8 minutes, or until the mixture comes to a boil. Reduce the heat to low. Cover the pan and cook for 15 minutes, or until tender. Remove from the heat.

3. While the rice cooks, prep the vegetables for the week:

   ☐ *Dice 2 yellow onions, and divide into 3 (½-cup) portions.*

   ☐ *Rinse and dice enough celery to divide into 2 (½-cup) portions.*

   ☐ *Mince enough garlic to measure 1 tablespoon.*

   ☐ *Slice 8 ounces cremini mushrooms.*

4. Preheat the oven to 350°F. Line a sheet pan with parchment paper.

5. Toast the pecans. Spread 1 cup chopped pecans out in a single layer on the prepared sheet pan. Transfer the sheet pan to the oven, and bake, stirring every 3 minutes, for 5 to 10 minutes, or until browned. Remove from the oven. Let cool.

6. Cook the bacon. In a large skillet, cook 12 bacon slices (or 8 slices if omitting from the quiche) over medium heat, turning every 2 to 3 minutes, for 7 to 10 minutes, or until they reach your desired crispness. Remove from the heat. Transfer to paper towels to drain and cool. Crumble the bacon.

7. Prepare the Crustless Broccoli Quiche (page 19) as directed. Let cool for 20 minutes. Tightly wrap the pan in aluminum foil, or put the quiche in an airtight container. Refrigerate for up to 4 days, or freeze for up to 2 months.

8. Prepare the Savory Bacon and Cheddar Pancakes (page 20) as directed. Let cool for 10 minutes. Place a sheet of wax paper or parchment paper between each pancake before putting it in a gallon-size freezer bag. Refrigerate for up to 5 days, or freeze for up to 2 months. Divide ½ cup maple syrup among 4 (1-ounce) containers for individual servings. Refrigerate for up to 1 year. Wrap 4 tablespoons butter (if using) in wax paper, and refrigerate for up to 3 months.

9. Prepare the Cranberry and Pecan Chicken Salad (page 21) as directed. Put the salad in an airtight container, or if making sandwiches, tightly wrap in aluminum foil or plastic storage bags. Refrigerate for up to 5 days. Freezing salads containing mayonnaise is not recommended because the ingredients will separate.

10. Prepare the Shrimp and Mushroom Pilaf (page 22) as directed. Let cool for 10 minutes. Put the pilaf in an airtight container. Refrigerate for up to 3 days, or freeze for up to 3 months.

Crustless Broccoli Quiche

PREP TIME: 15 MINUTES • COOK TIME: 35 TO 40 MINUTES

Although quiche originated in France, the word "quiche" is derived from "kuchen," the German word for cake. This quiche is naturally gluten-free, thanks to the lack of crust. **SERVES 4**

Nonstick cooking spray, for coating the pie pan

1 tablespoon salted butter

½ cup diced onion

1 (10-ounce) package chopped frozen broccoli

1 (15-ounce) container full-fat cottage cheese

4 large eggs, beaten

½ cup shredded mild Cheddar cheese

1 teaspoon garlic powder

½ teaspoon sea salt

¼ teaspoon freshly ground black pepper

4 bacon slices, cooked, drained, and crumbled (optional)

1. Preheat the oven to 350°F. Line a 9-inch pie pan with parchment paper, and coat with cooking spray.

2. In a large skillet, melt the butter over medium heat.

3. Add the onion and broccoli. Cook, stirring frequently, for 5 to 7 minutes, or until soft and the onion is translucent. Remove from the heat.

4. In a medium bowl, stir together the cottage cheese, eggs, Cheddar cheese, garlic powder, salt, pepper, and bacon (if using).

5. To make the filling, add the onion and broccoli mixture. Stir to combine.

6. Pour the filling into the prepared pie pan.

7. Transfer the pie pan to the oven, and bake for 25 to 30 minutes, or until a knife inserted into the center comes out clean. Remove from the oven. Let cool for 20 minutes.

STORAGE: Tightly wrap the pan in aluminum foil, or put the quiche in an airtight container. Refrigerate for up to 4 days, or freeze for up to 2 months.

THAWING AND REHEATING: Thaw in the refrigerator overnight. To reheat individual slices, cover with a damp paper towel. Microwave on high power for 30 seconds. Heat for 15 more seconds, if needed.

SUBSTITUTION TIP: Try cauliflower, spinach, or asparagus instead of broccoli.

Per Serving: Calories: 338; Total fat: 23g; Saturated fat: 12g; Protein: 23g; Total carbs: 10g; Fiber: 3g; Sugar: 5g; Sodium: 854mg

Savory Bacon and Cheddar Pancakes

PREP TIME: 20 MINUTES • COOK TIME: 20 MINUTES

These pancakes blend traditional comfort foods into a savory new combination. They are delicious served with a maple or fruit syrup, a drizzle of honey, and a pat of butter. SERVES 4

1⅔ cups all-purpose gluten-free one-to-one baking flour

½ teaspoon sea salt

1 teaspoon baking soda

1 teaspoon dried chives or 1 tablespoon minced fresh chives

2 large eggs, beaten

2 cups low-fat buttermilk

1 cup shredded mild Cheddar cheese

8 bacon slices, cooked, drained, and crumbled

Nonstick cooking spray, for coating the skillet

½ cup maple syrup

4 tablespoons (½ stick) salted butter (optional)

1. In a small bowl, whisk together the flour, salt, baking soda, and chives to combine.

2. In a large bowl, whisk together the eggs and buttermilk to blend.

3. To make the batter, add the flour mixture to the egg mixture. Stir to combine. Stir in the Cheddar cheese and bacon just until blended. The batter will be lumpy.

4. Heat a medium skillet over medium heat, and coat with cooking spray.

5. Making 1 pancake at a time, add ¾ cup of the batter, and cook for 2 to 3 minutes. Flip, and cook for 1 to 2 minutes, or until the pancake is firm. Continue with the remaining batter, coating the skillet with cooking spray before each pancake. Transfer to a plate. This should make 4 large pancakes. Turn off the heat. Let cool for 10 minutes.

6. Serve the pancakes with the maple syrup and butter (if using).

STORAGE: Place a sheet of wax paper or parchment paper between each pancake before putting it in a gallon-size freezer bag. Refrigerate for up to 5 days, or freeze for up to 2 months.

THAWING AND REHEATING: Thawed pancakes can be reheated in 30-second intervals.

Per Serving: Calories: 601; Total fat: 22g; Saturated fat: 10g; Protein: 26g; Total carbs: 74g; Fiber: 1g; Sugar: 32g; Sodium: 1,312mg

Cranberry and Pecan Chicken Salad

PREP TIME: 20 MINUTES • COOK TIME: 10 MINUTES

This creamy salad is a hit during any season. It can be served alone or made into sandwiches. Either way, you'll appreciate the sweet and savory blend of flavors. **SERVES 4**

1 pound boneless, skinless chicken breasts, cooked and diced

1 cup dried cranberries

½ cup diced onion

½ cup diced celery

½ teaspoon sea salt

½ teaspoon freshly ground black pepper

½ cup full-fat mayonnaise

½ cup crumbled goat cheese

1 cup chopped toasted pecans

1 loaf gluten-free bread, sliced

1. In a large bowl, stir together the chicken, dried cranberries, onion, celery, salt, and pepper.

2. Stir in the mayonnaise.

3. Fold in the goat cheese and pecans.

4. For sandwiches, spread ¾ cup of the chicken salad on a piece of bread. Top with another slice of bread.

STORAGE: Put the salad in an airtight container, or tightly wrap sandwiches in aluminum foil or plastic storage bags. Refrigerate for up to 5 days. Freezing salads containing mayonnaise is not recommended because the ingredients will separate.

SUBSTITUTION TIP: Easy swaps here include Greek yogurt for the mayonnaise, walnuts for the pecans, and golden raisins for the cranberries.

- -

Per Serving (4 bread slices): Calories: 922; Fat: 56g; Saturated fat: 9g; Protein: 37g; Total carbs: 75g; Fiber: 15g; Sugar: 24g; Sodium: 960mg

- -

Per Serving (2 bread slices): Calories: 772; Fat: 50g; Saturated fat: 8g; Protein: 34g; Total carbs: 53g; Fiber: 10g; Sugar: 23g; Sodium: 780mg

Shrimp and Mushroom Pilaf

PREP TIME: 15 MINUTES • COOK TIME: 10 MINUTES

Seafood lovers will rejoice at how easy it is to prepare this dish. Forkfuls of fluffy rice pair wonderfully with lightly sautéed, seasoned shrimp; plump, juicy mushrooms; and a blend of onion, celery, and garlic. SERVES 4

¼ **cup extra-virgin olive oil**

½ **cup diced onion**

½ **cup diced celery**

1 **tablespoon minced garlic**

1 **(8-ounce) container cremini mushrooms, sliced**

1 **pound frozen medium shrimp, peeled, deveined, tails removed**

1 **teaspoon Italian seasoning**

½ **teaspoon freshly ground black pepper**

3 **cups cooked long-grain white rice**

1. In a large skillet, heat the oil over medium heat.

2. Add the onion, celery, garlic, and mushrooms. Cook, stirring often, for 5 to 7 minutes, or until the onion is tender and translucent.

3. Add the shrimp, Italian seasoning, and pepper. Cook, stirring constantly, for about 3 minutes, or until the shrimp are opaque. Remove from the heat.

4. Stir in the rice. Let cool for 10 minutes.

STORAGE: Put in an airtight container. Refrigerate for up to 3 days, or freeze for up to 3 months.

THAWING AND REHEATING: Thaw in the refrigerator overnight. To reheat, put in a microwave-safe dish, add 1 tablespoon water, and cover with a paper towel. Microwave on 50 percent power in 30-second intervals, stirring after each, until warm.

SUBSTITUTION TIP: Replace the shrimp with 2 cups diced cooked chicken, pork, or steak.

INGREDIENT TIP: Choose fresher shrimp by heading to the freezer section. These shrimp are usually frozen as soon as they're brought onto the boat. The shrimp at the seafood counter have usually been frozen, then thawed for purchase.

Per Serving: Calories: 382; Total fat: 15g; Saturated fat: 2g; Protein: 21g; Total carbs: 40g; Fiber: 2g; Sugar: 2g; Sodium: 710mg

SUMMER MENU:
Four-Recipe Meal Prep

Now that you've got the hang of meal prep, I've added a recipe containing a few more ingredients. Don't worry, it still comes together in a snap. With soaring temperatures outside, spending time in a hot kitchen is a drag. All these recipes are designed to beat the heat. From a cool, creamy smoothie to start the day to a light pasta dish that's perfect served with a glass of wine or a sparkling cider, this prep is chock-full of fresh summer fruits and vegetables. We'll also prepare Italian Dressing (page 182) to serve with the salad. Read the recipes before your shopping trip to be sure you have the required spices. Simple swaps include green olives for black olives, honey or agave to replace sugar, Italian-style diced tomatoes for regular tomatoes, or a rice of choice to replace the pasta.

SUMMER MENU:
Four-Recipe Meal Prep Shopping List

PRODUCE

Basil (1 large bunch; need 1 cup leaves)

Bell peppers, green (2)

Blackberries (1 pint)

Garlic (1 head)

Mixed greens (1 [1-pound] package)

Onions, yellow (2)

Raspberries (1 pint)

Squash, yellow (1)

Strawberries (1 pint)

Tomatoes, large (4)

Zucchini (1)

DAIRY AND EGGS

Cheese, feta, crumbled (1 [5-ounce] container)

Milk, low-fat (1 pint)

Yogurt, low-fat, vanilla (1 [1-pound] container)

MEAT

Beef, steak, sirloin, boneless (1 pound)

Chicken, breasts, boneless, skinless (1½ pounds)

CANNED AND BOTTLED

Olives, black, sliced (1 [15-ounce] can)

Tomatoes, diced (1 [14½-ounce] can)

PANTRY

Pasta, gluten-free (1 [12-ounce] package)

CHECK YOUR PANTRY FOR . . .

Balsamic vinegar, black peppercorns, celery seed, distilled white vinegar, dried basil, dried oregano, dried parsley, dried thyme, extra-virgin olive oil, garlic powder, Italian seasoning, nonstick cooking spray, onion powder, red pepper flakes, sea salt, sugar or honey

Weekly Meal Chart

	BREAKFAST	LUNCH	DINNER
DAY 1	Very Berry Smoothie	Steak Salad	Steak Salad
DAY 2	Very Berry Smoothie	Steak Salad	Tomato-Basil Pasta
DAY 3		Chicken with Summer Squash	Steak Salad
DAY 4	Very Berry Smoothie	Steak Salad	Tomato-Basil Pasta
DAY 5	Very Berry Smoothie	Tomato-Basil Pasta	Chicken with Summer Squash

STEP-BY-STEP PREP

1. Prep the vegetables:

   ☐ *Chop 2 yellow onions and divide into 2 (¾-cup) portions.*

   ☐ *Thinly slice 1 zucchini.*

   ☐ *Thinly slice 1 yellow squash.*

   ☐ *Chop 4 tomatoes.*

   ☐ *Seed and chop 2 green bell peppers and divide into 2 (¾-cup) portions.*

   ☐ *Mince 1 cup fresh basil leaves.*

   ☐ *Mince enough garlic to measure 3 tablespoons.*

   ☐ *Hull 1 pint strawberries.*

2. Dice 1½ pounds boneless, skinless chicken breasts. Prepare the Chicken with Summer Squash (page 27) as directed. Let cool for 20 minutes. Put in an airtight container, and refrigerate for up to 4 days, or freeze for up to 3 months.

3. Make the Italian Dressing (page 182) for the Steak Salad (page 28).

4. Cut 1 pound sirloin steak into 1-inch strips. Prepare the Steak Salad (page 28) as directed. Let the steak-vegetable mixture cool for 15 minutes. Put individual salads in airtight containers. Refrigerate for up to 4 days. Although the steak mixture can be frozen for up to 3 months, prepared salads should not be frozen. Put 1 tablespoon prepared dressing in each of 4 (1-ounce) containers. Refrigerate for up to 1 week.

5. Cook 12 ounces gluten-free pasta for 4 minutes less than the package directions indicate. Drain, and rinse with cool water.

6. Prepare the Tomato-Basil Pasta (page 29) as directed. Put in an airtight container, and refrigerate for up to 5 days, or freeze for up to 2 months. See the ingredient tip (page 29).

7. Make the Very Berry Smoothie (page 30) as directed. To make individual servings, portion the smoothies into 4 (8-ounce) Mason jars. Seal tightly. Refrigerate for up to 4 days, or freeze for up to 3 months.

Chicken with Summer Squash

PREP TIME: 20 MINUTES • COOK TIME: 30 TO 35 MINUTES

Fresh summer vegetables are the star of this dish. Excess garden zucchini gets a new life, sliced thinly, paired with yellow squash, and served with chunks of chicken and diced tomato. **SERVES 4**

Nonstick cooking spray, for coating the baking dish

¼ cup extra-virgin olive oil

1½ pounds boneless, skinless, chicken breasts (about 2)

¾ cup chopped green bell pepper

¾ cup chopped yellow onion

1 zucchini, thinly sliced

1 yellow squash, thinly sliced

1 tablespoon minced garlic

1 (14½-ounce) can diced tomatoes

1 tablespoon Italian seasoning

1 teaspoon sea salt

½ teaspoon freshly ground black pepper

1. Preheat the oven to 400°F. Coat a 9-by-9-inch baking dish with cooking spray.

2. In a large skillet, combine the oil and chicken. Cook over medium heat for 6 minutes, flipping halfway through, or until browned. Remove from the heat.

3. In a large bowl, stir together the bell pepper, onion, zucchini, squash, garlic, tomatoes, Italian seasoning, salt, and pepper until blended.

4. Pour the vegetables into the prepared baking dish. Top with the chicken.

5. Transfer the baking dish to the oven, and bake for 20 to 25 minutes, or until the chicken reaches an internal temperature of 165°F and the vegetables are tender when pierced with a fork. Remove from the oven. Let cool for 20 minutes.

STORAGE: Put in an airtight container. Refrigerate for up to 4 days, or freeze for up to 3 months.

THAWING AND REHEATING: Thaw in the refrigerator overnight. To reheat individual servings, put on a microwave-safe plate. Microwave on high power for 45 seconds. Stir and heat for 15 to 30 more seconds, if needed.

Per Serving: Calories: 367; Total fat: 19g; Saturated fat: 3g; Protein: 40g; Total carbs: 9g; Fiber: 3g; Sugar: 6g; Sodium: 797mg

Steak Salad

PREP TIME: 20 MINUTES • COOK TIME: 5 TO 10 MINUTES

You get a variety of flavors in this salad. From the earthy taste of feta to the tang of homemade Italian dressing, this dish will have you craving salad for lunch. SERVES 4

¼ cup extra-virgin olive oil

¾ cup chopped green
  bell pepper

¾ cup chopped yellow onion

1 tablespoon minced garlic

1 pound boneless sirloin
  steak, cut into 1-inch-
  thick strips

1 (15-ounce) can sliced black
  olives, drained

1 (1-pound) package
  mixed greens

¼ cup crumbled feta cheese

¼ cup Italian Dressing
  (page 182)

1. In a large skillet, combine the oil, bell pepper, onion, garlic, and steak. Cook over medium heat for 5 to 7 minutes, or until the onion is tender and translucent and the steak is no longer pink. Remove from the heat. Transfer to a large bowl. Let cool for 15 minutes. Using paper towels, pat dry, making sure no moisture remains.

2. Stir in the olives.

3. To make individual salads, put ¼ cup of the steak mixture in each of 4 (16-ounce) airtight containers.

4. Top with 1 cup of mixed greens and 1 tablespoon of feta cheese.

5. Divide the dressing among 4 (1-ounce) containers.

6. Serve the salads with the dressing.

STORAGE: Refrigerate the salads for up to 4 days. The steak mixture alone may be frozen in an airtight container for up to 3 months, but the prepared salads should not be frozen because the greens will become mushy. Refrigerate the dressing for up to 1 week.

THAWING AND REHEATING: Thaw the steak mixture in the refrigerator overnight. You can heat the steak or leave it cold. To heat individual servings, put on a microwave-safe plate. Microwave on high power for 30 seconds.

Per Serving: Calories: 630; Total fat: 52g; Saturated fat: 12g; Protein: 27g; Total carbs: 16g; Fiber: 5g; Sugar: 5g; Sodium: 829mg

Tomato-Basil Pasta

PREP TIME: 20 MINUTES

This simple dish takes minutes to prepare and showcases fresh, ripe summer tomatoes. Although the tomato-basil mixture is delicious served with pasta, it can be served alone as an appetizer or salad. SERVES 4

1½ **cups extra-virgin olive oil**

¼ **cup distilled white vinegar**

1 **tablespoon minced garlic**

1½ **teaspoons sea salt**

½ **teaspoon freshly ground black pepper**

4 **large tomatoes, chopped**

1 **cup fresh basil leaves, minced**

1 **(12-ounce) package gluten-free pasta, cooked for 4 minutes less than the package directions indicate**

¼ **cup crumbled feta cheese (optional)**

1. In a large bowl, whisk together the oil, vinegar, garlic, salt, and pepper.

2. Using a paper towel, pat the tomatoes dry.

3. Add the tomatoes and basil to the bowl. Stir until blended.

4. Stir in the pasta.

5. Top with the cheese (if using).

STORAGE: Put in an airtight container. Refrigerate for up to 5 days, or freeze for up to 2 months.

THAWING AND REHEATING: Thaw in the refrigerator overnight. To heat individual servings, put the pasta in a microwave-safe bowl. Microwave on high power for 1 minute. Stir and heat for 30 more seconds, if needed.

SUBSTITUTION TIP: Simple swaps for this recipe include red-wine vinegar or balsamic vinegar instead of white and spinach instead of basil. Good mix-ins include chopped yellow onion, green bell pepper, and black olives. One cup chopped prosciutto can also be added.

INGREDIENT TIP: Gluten-free pasta can become mushy when frozen. To help prevent this, undercook the pasta by 4 minutes. Make sure the pasta is completely covered by sauce or stored separately before freezing.

Per Serving: Calories: 1,065; Total fat: 83g; Saturated fat: 12g; Protein: 8g; Total carbs: 74g; Fiber: 5g; Sugar: 5g; Sodium: 883mg

Very Berry Smoothie

PREP TIME: 10 MINUTES

This smoothie delivers a burst of berry flavor with each creamy sip. A welcome pick-me-up in the morning, it's a great way to use any extra fruit you have in the refrigerator or freezer. **SERVES 4**

16 ounces low-fat vanilla yogurt

2 cups low-fat milk

1 pint fresh raspberries

1 pint fresh strawberries, hulled

1 pint fresh blackberries

½ cup sugar

12 ice cubes

In a high-speed blender, combine the yogurt, milk, raspberries, strawberries, blackberries, sugar, and ice. Pulse for 10 to 15 seconds, or until the berries are pureed.

STORAGE: Put in an airtight container or tightly sealed jars. Refrigerate for up to 4 days, or freeze for up to 3 months.

THAWING AND REHEATING: Thaw in the refrigerator overnight. Stir before serving.

SUBSTITUTION TIP: Replace the fresh berries and the ice cubes with 1 (32-ounce) package frozen triple-berry blend (strawberries, blueberries, and blackberries). If you have any leftover fresh berries and yogurt, they can be used in Triple-Berry Parfaits (page 195).

INGREDIENT TIP: Have an abundance of berries? Freeze them. Wash strawberries under running water, pat dry, remove the green stems, and put on a sheet pan. Freeze for 1 to 2 hours, or until firm, and transfer to an airtight freezer-safe container. Keep frozen for up to 1 year.

To freeze blackberries, blueberries, or raspberries, place the berries in a bowl of cool water to rinse. Drain, and pat dry. Remove the leaves and stems from blackberries. Place the berries on a sheet pan, and freeze for about 1 hour, or until firm. Transfer to an airtight freezer-safe container and keep frozen for up to 1 year.

- -

Per Serving: Calories: 392; Total fat: 5g; Saturated fat: 3g; Protein: 13g; Total carbs: 79g; Fiber: 8g; Sugar: 69g; Sodium: 142mg

FALL MENU:
Four-Recipe Meal Prep

F all brings cozy warm dishes to combat the nip in the air, like Pasta e Fagioli (page 37) and Sheet Pan Pork Chops with Fall Vegetables (page 35). Pork chops freeze especially well. When you prepare the sheet pan pork chops, purchase extra chops, season, and bake without the vegetables, if desired. Serve them with a side of mashed potatoes or rice for variety. Bake extra sweet potatoes to serve as an easy lunch or side dish. You might have noticed some recipe ingredients are only available in larger quantities than used in the prep. Any leftover Cheddar cheese can be added to the fried rice. Leftover cooked or raw vegetables can be added to soups, and leftover cooked pasta can be added to soup a few minutes before serving. The possibilities are endless.

FALL MENU:
Four-Recipe Meal Prep Shopping List

PRODUCE
Bell pepper, green (1)
Brussels sprouts (1 pound)
Cabbage, green (1 head)
Carrots (2)
Garlic (1 head)
Mushrooms, cremini (1 [8-ounce] package)
Onions, yellow (2)
Sweet potatoes (4)

DAIRY AND EGGS
Butter, salted (8 ounces)
Cheese, Cheddar, sharp, shredded
   (1 [8-ounce] bag)
Eggs, large (1 half dozen)
Milk, 2 percent (1 pint)

MEAT
Beef, ground, 80/20 (1 pound)
Pork, bone-in chops (4 [8-ounce])

FROZEN FOOD
Broccoli, chopped (1 [10-ounce] package)
Peas and carrots (1 [10-ounce] package)

CANNED AND BOTTLED
Broth, vegetable (2 [14½-ounce] containers)
Chickpeas (1 [15-ounce] can)
Soy sauce or tamari, gluten-free
   (1 [10-ounce] bottle)
Tomatoes, Italian-style, diced
   (1 [28-ounce] can)
Water chestnuts, sliced (1 [8-ounce] can)

PANTRY
Flour, all-purpose gluten-free one-to-one
   baking (1 [16-ounce] package)
Elbow macaroni, gluten-free (1 [12-ounce]
   package)
Pecans, chopped (¼ cup)
Rice, basmati (1 [16-ounce] package)

CHECK YOUR PANTRY FOR . . .
Baking powder, black peppercorns, cayenne pepper, dried basil,
extra-virgin olive oil, garlic powder,
ground cinnamon, ground nutmeg,
Italian seasoning, nonstick cooking
spray, onion powder, paprika, sea
salt, sugar

Weekly Meal Chart

	BREAKFAST	LUNCH	DINNER
DAY 1	Sweet Potato Muffins	Vegetable Fried Rice	Sheet Pan Pork Chops with Fall Vegetables
DAY 2	Sweet Potato Muffins	Pasta e Fagioli	Vegetable Fried Rice
DAY 3	Sweet Potato Muffins	Sheet Pan Pork Chops with Fall Vegetables	Pasta e Fagioli
DAY 4	Sweet Potato Muffins	Sheet Pan Pork Chops with Fall Vegetables	Pasta e Fagioli
DAY 5	Sweet Potato Muffins	Vegetable Fried Rice	Sheet Pan Pork Chops with Fall Vegetables

STEP-BY-STEP PREP

1. Cook the sweet potatoes. Using a fork, prick 2 sweet potatoes 5 times each. Microwave on high power, checking every 5 minutes, for 15 to 20 minutes, or until soft. Let cool for 10 minutes, then peel and mash.

2. While the sweet potatoes cook, prep the vegetables for the week:

   ☐ *Trim and halve 1 pound Brussels sprouts.*

   ☐ *Finely chop enough cabbage to measure 2 cups.*

   ☐ *Dice 2 yellow onions, and divide into 2 (1-cup) portions.*

   ☐ *Seed and dice 1 green bell pepper.*

   ☐ *Mince enough garlic to measure 2 tablespoons.*

   ☐ *Peel 2 carrots and cut into ½-inch-thick slices.*

   ☐ *Slice 8 ounces cremini mushrooms.*

   ☐ *Dice 2 sweet potatoes.*

3. Cook the rice. In a large saucepan, combine 1¾ cups water and 1 cup basmati rice. Bring to a boil over medium heat. Reduce the heat to low. Stir, cover the pan, and simmer for 20 minutes, or until fluffy and tender. Remove from the heat. Let cool for 10 minutes.

4. Preheat the oven to 400°F. Prepare the Sheet Pan Pork Chops with Fall Vegetables (page 35) as directed. Let cool for 20 minutes. Package the meat and vegetables in divided airtight containers. Refrigerate for up to 5 days, or freeze for up to 3 months.

5. Cook 2 cups elbow macaroni for 4 minutes less than the package directions indicate. Drain.

6. Cook the ground beef. In a medium skillet, cook the ground beef over medium heat, stirring occasionally, for 7 to 10 minutes, or until no longer pink. Remove from the heat. Prepare the Pasta e Fagioli (page 37) as directed. Let cool for 20 minutes. Store the soup and cooked pasta in separate airtight freezer-safe containers. Spoon 1 tablespoon Cheddar cheese into each of 4 (1-ounce) containers. The soup and pasta can be refrigerated for up to 5 days or frozen for up to 3 months. The cheese can be refrigerated for up to 1 week or frozen for up to 6 months.

7. Prepare the Sweet Potato Muffins (page 38) as directed. Let cool for 20 minutes. Put in an airtight container or resealable bag. Store at room temperature for up to 3 days, refrigerate for up to 5 days, or freeze for up to 3 months.

8. Prepare the Vegetable Fried Rice (page 40) as directed. Let cool for 20 minutes. Put in an airtight container. Refrigerate for up to 5 days, or freeze up to 3 months.

Sheet Pan Pork Chops with Fall Vegetables

PREP TIME: 20 MINUTES • COOK TIME: 35 MINUTES

Fix it and (almost) forget it! That's the simplicity of this sheet pan recipe. Succulent pork chops and crisp vegetables are topped with a Creole-type seasoning and baked to a golden brown. **SERVES 4**

For the pork chop seasoning

½ **cup extra-virgin olive oil**

2 **teaspoons paprika**

2 **teaspoons onion powder**

2 **teaspoons garlic powder**

1 **teaspoon sea salt**

1 **teaspoon freshly ground black pepper**

1 **teaspoon cayenne pepper**

For the pork chops and vegetables

1 **pound Brussels sprouts, trimmed and halved**

2 **carrots, thinly sliced**

2 **sweet potatoes, diced**

4 **(8-ounce) bone-in pork chops**

To make the pork chop seasoning

1. In a small bowl, stir together the oil, paprika, onion powder, garlic powder, salt, black pepper, and cayenne.

To make the pork chops and vegetables

2. Preheat the oven to 400°F. Line a large sheet pan with parchment paper.

3. In a large bowl, combine the Brussels sprouts, carrots, and sweet potatoes.

4. Add half of the seasoning, and using your clean hands, mix to coat.

5. Put the pork chops on the prepared sheet pan, and sprinkle with the remaining seasoning.

6. Spread the Brussels sprouts and sweet potatoes around the chops.

7. Transfer the sheet pan to the oven, and bake for 10 minutes.

8. Add the carrots to the sheet pan, and bake for 10 minutes.

9. Flip the chops, and stir the vegetables. Bake for 10 to 15 minutes, or until the chops reach an internal temperature of 145°F. The vegetables should be crispy on the outside and tender on the inside. Remove from the oven.

STORAGE: Put in airtight containers. Refrigerate for up to 5 days, or freeze for up to 3 months.

CONTINUED ⋯→

THAWING AND REHEATING: Thaw in the refrigerator overnight. To reheat individual servings, put on a microwave-safe dish, and loosely cover with a paper towel. Microwave on 50 percent power for 45 seconds. Stir the vegetables, and heat for 30 more seconds.

SUBSTITUTION TIP: Brussels sprouts can be replaced with diced Russet potatoes, turnips, parsnips, or cauliflower.

PREPARATION TIP: Sheet pan wisdom says be careful not to overcrowd the pan, which causes the ingredients to steam instead of bake. You may need to use 2 sheet pans to provide ample space.

Per Serving: Calories: 659; Total fat: 43g; Saturated fat: 9g; Protein: 40g; Total carbs: 29g; Fiber: 8g; Sugar: 7g; Sodium: 763mg

Pasta e Fagioli

PREP TIME: 20 MINUTES • COOK TIME: 40 MINUTES

A bowl of this nourishing soup is sure to warm both your heart and stomach. Ground beef, cabbage, and pasta make this a hearty soup. SERVES 4

4 tablespoons (½ stick) salted butter

1 cup diced yellow onion

1 cup diced green bell pepper

1 tablespoon minced garlic

1 (28-ounce) can Italian-seasoned diced tomatoes

2 cups vegetable broth

2 teaspoons Italian seasoning

1 teaspoon dried basil

1 teaspoon sea salt

1 teaspoon freshly ground black pepper

2 cups finely chopped cabbage

1 (15-ounce) can chickpeas, drained and rinsed

1 pound 80/20 ground beef, cooked, drained, and crumbled

2 cups gluten-free elbow macaroni, cooked for 4 minutes less than the package directions indicate

½ cup shredded sharp Cheddar cheese

1. In a large saucepan or Dutch oven, melt the butter over medium heat.

2. Add the onion, bell pepper, and garlic. Cook for 5 to 7 minutes, or until the onion is tender and translucent.

3. Stir in the tomatoes, broth, Italian seasoning, basil, salt, pepper, cabbage, chickpeas, and beef. Bring to a boil, stirring often.

4. Reduce the heat to low. Cover the pan, and simmer, stirring often, for 20 minutes, or until the mixture has slightly thickened. Remove from the heat.

STORAGE: Refrigerate the soup and cooked pasta in separate airtight freezer-safe containers for up to 5 days, or freeze for up to 3 months. The cheese can be refrigerated for up to 1 week or frozen for up to 6 months.

THAWING AND REHEATING: Thaw in the refrigerator overnight. To heat individual servings, put the soup in a microwave-safe dish, and cover with a paper towel. Microwave on high power for 30 seconds. Stir and heat for 15 to 30 more seconds. Put the pasta in a microwave-safe bowl, and microwave on high power for 15 seconds. Stir the hot pasta into the soup. Sprinkle with cheese before serving.

SUBSTITUTION TIP: Replace the ground beef with Italian sausage and the vegetable broth with beef broth.

Per Serving: Calories: 748; Total fat: 42g; Saturated fat: 19g; Protein: 36g; Total carbs: 58g; Fiber: 13g; Sugar: 13g; Sodium: 855mg

Sweet Potato Muffins

PREP TIME: 20 MINUTES • COOK TIME: 20 TO 25 MINUTES

Sweet potatoes are a vegetable powerhouse—packed with beta-carotene, vitamins, potassium, and iron. They add moistness to these muffins, and the cinnamon and nutmeg make them taste almost like sweet potato pie. MAKES 18 MUFFINS

Nonstick cooking spray, for coating the muffin tins

8 tablespoons (1 stick) salted butter, melted

1¼ cups sugar

2 large eggs, beaten

1½ cups all-purpose gluten-free one-to-one baking flour

2 teaspoons baking powder

1 teaspoon ground cinnamon

¼ teaspoon sea salt

¼ teaspoon ground nutmeg

1 cup 2 percent milk

2 sweet potatoes, cooked, peeled, and mashed

¼ cup chopped pecans

1. Preheat the oven to 400°F. Coat 2 (12-cup) muffin tins with cooking spray.

2. In a large bowl, using a handheld mixer, cream the butter and sugar on medium speed for about 2 minutes, or until fluffy.

3. Add the eggs, and mix until blended.

4. In a medium bowl, stir together the flour, baking powder, cinnamon, salt, and nutmeg until blended.

5. To make the batter, alternate adding the flour mixture and milk to the butter mixture, blending after each addition.

6. Turn off the mixer. Stir in the sweet potatoes and pecans.

7. Spoon ⅓ cup of the batter into each prepared muffin cup.

8. Transfer the muffin tins to the oven, and bake for 15 to 20 minutes, or until a knife inserted into the center of a muffin comes out clean. Remove from the oven.

STORAGE: Store in an airtight container or resealable bag at room temperature for up to 3 days, refrigerate for up to 5 days, or freeze for up to 3 months.

THAWING AND REHEATING: To heat a frozen muffin, put it on a microwave-safe dish or paper towel. Microwave on high power for 30 to 45 seconds. The muffins can also be thawed at room temperature for 2 to 3 hours.

SUBSTITUTION TIP: Replace the pecans with walnuts, or add ½ cup chocolate chips.

INGREDIENT TIP: To choose the perfect sweet potatoes, look for medium ones, which tend to be more tender than large ones. Always choose firm, smooth sweet potatoes.

Per Serving (2 muffins): Calories: 352; Total fat: 14g; Saturated fat: 7g; Protein: 5g; Total carbs: 52g; Fiber: 2g; Sugar: 31g; Sodium: 265mg

Vegetable Fried Rice

PREP TIME: 20 MINUTES • COOK TIME: 20 MINUTES

Tamari is the Japanese version of soy sauce, made as a by-product of miso and rarely containing wheat. So it is naturally gluten-free, but check the label to be sure. This dish gets an unexpected crunch from water chestnuts and broccoli. **SERVES 4**

4 tablespoons (½ stick) salted butter, divided

2 large eggs, beaten

1 cup diced yellow onion

1 tablespoon minced garlic

1 (10-ounce) package frozen chopped broccoli

1 (8-ounce) can sliced water chestnuts, drained

1 (8-ounce) container cremini mushrooms, sliced

1 teaspoon sea salt

1 teaspoon freshly ground black pepper

1 (10-ounce) package frozen peas and carrots

1 cup vegetable broth

3 cups cooked basmati rice

½ cup gluten-free soy sauce or tamari

1. In a large skillet, melt 2 tablespoons of butter over medium heat.

2. Add the eggs, and cook, stirring often, for 2 minutes. Remove from the heat. Transfer to a plate.

3. To the skillet, add the remaining 2 tablespoons of butter, the onion, garlic, broccoli, water chestnuts, mushrooms, salt, and pepper. Cook, stirring often, for about 7 minutes, or until the onion is translucent.

4. Add the peas and carrots and broth. Cook for 5 to 7 minutes, or until the vegetables are tender when pierced with a fork.

5. Return the eggs to the skillet.

6. Stir in the rice and soy sauce. Cook, stirring constantly, for 1 minute, or until heated through. Remove from the heat.

STORAGE: Put in an airtight container. Refrigerate for up to 5 days, or freeze up to 3 months.

THAWING AND REHEATING: Thaw in the refrigerator overnight. To reheat individual servings, put the rice in a microwave-safe dish, add 1 tablespoon water, and loosely cover with a paper towel, venting one side. Microwave on high power in 30-second intervals, stirring after each, or until warm.

INGREDIENT TIP: Tired of rice? Try buckwheat. In a large saucepan, combine 2 cups water and 1 cup raw buckwheat. Bring to a boil over medium heat. Cover the pan, reduce the heat to low, and simmer for 10 minutes.

WINTER MENU:
Four-Recipe Meal Prep

F rigid temperatures, overcast days, and long, dark nights. It's no wonder we crave filling foods in winter. This menu delivers on that promise with a corn and salsa–stuffed breakfast tortilla, a creamy soup, and herbed chicken with noodles. Shop your pantry first, and use any type of rice you prefer, millet, or buckwheat to replace cauliflower "rice," or substitute kidney beans for the black beans. Leftover cooked rice may be added to the soup or the burritos. Any leftover tortillas can be used to make Spicy Tortilla Chips (page 189). Now that you've gotten the hang of meal prep, you might want to invest in another kitchen tool. If you are ready to expand your cookware, a Dutch oven is a good choice because of its versatility. Made either of heavy metal or ceramic, these pots have a tight-fitting lid and can be used on the stovetop and in the oven.

WINTER MENU:
Four-Recipe Meal Prep Shopping List

PRODUCE
Avocados (2)
Cauliflower (1 head)
Celery (1 bunch)
Cilantro (1 bunch)
Garlic (1 large head)
Limes (2)
Onions, yellow (2)

DAIRY AND EGGS
Butter, salted (8 ounces)
Cheese, Cheddar, sharp, shredded
   (1 [8-ounce] bag)
Eggs, large (1 dozen)
Milk, whole (1 pint)
Sour cream, full-fat (1 [8-ounce] container)

MEAT
Chicken, breasts, boneless, skinless
   (2 pounds; about 4 pieces)
Sausage, Italian (1 pound)

FROZEN FOOD
Broccoli, chopped (2 [10-ounce] packages)

CANNED AND BOTTLED
Beans, black (2 [15-ounce] cans)
Broth, vegetable (1 [32-ounce] container)
Corn, cream-style (1 [14½-ounce] can)
Salsa verde (1 [16-ounce] can or jar)

PANTRY
Bread crumbs, gluten-free (1 [9-ounce]
   container)
Rice, long-grain, white (1 [8-ounce] package)
Tortillas, flour, 8-inch, gluten-free
   (1 [6-count] package)

CHECK YOUR PANTRY FOR . . .
All-purpose gluten-free one-to-one
baking flour, bay leaves, black peppercorns, dried oregano, dried parsley
flakes, dried thyme, extra-virgin olive
oil, garlic powder, ground cumin, Italian seasoning, nonstick cooking spray,
paprika, sea salt

Weekly Meal Chart

	BREAKFAST	LUNCH	DINNER
DAY 1	Corn and Salsa Breakfast Burritos	Black Beans and Rice	Cheesy Broccoli and Sausage Soup
DAY 2	Corn and Salsa Breakfast Burritos	Crumb-Coated Chicken with Cauliflower "Rice"	Black Beans and Rice
DAY 3		Crumb-Coated Chicken with Cauliflower "Rice"	Cheesy Broccoli and Sausage Soup
DAY 4	Corn and Salsa Breakfast Burritos	Black Beans and Rice	Crumb-Coated Chicken with Cauliflower "Rice"
DAY 5	Corn and Salsa Breakfast Burritos	Cheesy Broccoli and Sausage Soup	Black Beans and Rice

STEP-BY-STEP-PREP

1. Cook the rice. In a large saucepan, combine 2 cups water and 1 cup long-grain white rice. Bring to a boil over high heat. Reduce the heat to low. Cover the pan, and simmer for 15 minutes, or until tender. Remove from the heat. Let rest for 10 minutes. Remove the rice, and wash the saucepan to use for the soup.

2. While the rice cooks, prep the vegetables for the week:

☐ *Chop 2 yellow onions.*

☐ *Chop enough celery to measure ½ cup.*

☐ *Mince enough garlic to measure 2 tablespoons.*

☐ *Finely chop enough cilantro to measure ½ cup.*

☐ *Juice enough limes to measure 2 tablespoons juice.*

☐ *"Rice" the cauliflower: Wash 1 head cauliflower, and*

remove the green leaves. Chop the cauliflower into large pieces. Using a cheese grater or box grater, shred the large pieces on the largest holes.

3. Cook the cauliflower. In a large skillet, heat 2 tablespoons olive oil over medium heat. Add 3 cups grated cauliflower. Cook, stirring often, for 5 minutes, or until tender and fluffy. Remove from the heat. Transfer to a plate, and wash the skillet.

4. Cook the sausage. In the same skillet, cook 1 pound Italian sausage over medium heat for 7 to 10 minutes, or until browned and no pink remains. Remove from the heat. Drain, and let cool. Crumble the sausage.

5. Prepare the Cheesy Broccoli and Sausage Soup (page 45) as directed. Let cool for 20 minutes. Pour into an airtight container, and refrigerate up to 4 days, or freeze for up to 3 months.

6. Prepare the Crumb-Coated Chicken with Cauliflower "Rice" (page 46) as directed. Let cool for 15 minutes. Spoon the cooked cauliflower rice into an airtight container. Place the chicken on top of the rice. Refrigerate for up to 3 days, or freeze up to 3 months.

7. Prepare the Black Beans and Rice (page 47) as directed. Let cool for 10 minutes. Package in an airtight container, and refrigerate for up to 5 days, or freeze for up to 3 months. Put 1 tablespoon sour cream in each of 4 (2-ounce) serving containers, and refrigerate for up to 1 week. Pat the chopped cilantro dry using a paper towel, and wrap in a fresh paper towel. Put in a storage bag, and squeeze out all the air. Refrigerate for up to 2 weeks. The avocado must be prepped just before serving.

8. Prepare the Corn and Salsa Breakfast Burritos (page 48) as directed. Let cool for 15 minutes. Wrap each burrito tightly in aluminum foil before putting in an airtight container. Refrigerate for up to 4 days, or freeze for up to 3 months. Prepare the cilantro as directed in step 7. The avocado must be prepped just before serving.

Cheesy Broccoli and Sausage Soup

PREP TIME: 20 MINUTES • COOK TIME: 40 MINUTES

This soup gets its creaminess from sharp Cheddar cheese and whole milk instead of the typical heavy cream. The Italian sausage offers a twist on traditional broccoli soup. SERVES 4

2 tablespoons salted butter, melted

2 (10-ounce) packages frozen chopped broccoli

½ cup chopped celery

½ cup chopped yellow onion

2 teaspoons dried parsley flakes

1 teaspoon sea salt

½ teaspoon freshly ground black pepper

2 cups vegetable broth

¼ cup all-purpose gluten-free one-to-one baking flour

2 cups whole milk, divided

1 pound Italian sausage, cooked, drained, and crumbled

1 cup shredded sharp Cheddar cheese

1. In a large saucepan, combine the butter, broccoli, celery, onion, parsley flakes, salt, pepper, and broth. Bring to a boil over medium heat, and cover the pan.

2. Reduce the heat to low. Simmer, stirring occasionally, for 10 minutes.

3. To make a slurry, in a small bowl, whisk together the flour and 1 cup of milk until dissolved.

4. Add the slurry to the soup, and stir until blended.

5. Stir in the remaining l cup of milk, and simmer, stirring occasionally, for 20 to 25 minutes, or until the soup thickens.

6. Stir in the sausage and Cheddar cheese. Cook, stirring, until the cheese melts and the sausage is warmed. Remove from the heat. Let cool for 20 minutes before storing.

STORAGE: Put in an airtight container. Refrigerate for up to 4 days, or freeze for up to 3 months.

THAWING AND REHEATING: Thaw in the refrigerator overnight. To reheat individual servings, put the soup in a microwave-safe bowl, and loosely cover using a paper towel. Microwave on high power for 30 seconds. Stir and heat for 15 to 30 more seconds. Stir before serving.

Per Serving: Calories: 711; Total fat: 51g; Saturated fat: 22g; Protein: 38g; Total carbs: 27g; Fiber: 5g; Sugar: 10g; Sodium: 1,634mg

NUT-FREE • SOY-FREE

Crumb-Coated Chicken with Cauliflower "Rice"

PREP TIME: 20 MINUTES • COOK TIME: 20 MINUTES

Tender, juicy chicken flavored with herbs and cheese gets an unexpected sidekick in this recipe—"rice" made from shredded cauliflower. Once you try it, you may never go back to ordinary rice. **SERVES 4**

Nonstick cooking spray, for coating the sheet pan

2 tablespoons salted butter, melted

1 large egg, beaten

1 cup gluten-free bread crumbs

1 teaspoon garlic powder

1 teaspoon Italian seasoning

½ teaspoon sea salt

½ teaspoon freshly ground black pepper

½ teaspoon paprika

½ cup shredded sharp Cheddar cheese

2 pounds boneless, skinless chicken breasts (about 4)

3 cups cauliflower rice, cooked (1 head cauliflower)

1. Preheat the oven to 350°F. Coat a sheet pan with cooking spray.

2. In a shallow bowl, stir together the butter and egg until combined.

3. In another shallow bowl, stir together the bread crumbs, garlic powder, Italian seasoning, salt, pepper, paprika, and cheese until combined.

4. One piece at a time, dip the chicken into the butter mixture, then in the crumb mixture.

5. Place the coated chicken in a single layer on the prepared sheet pan.

6. Transfer the sheet pan to the oven, and bake for 20 minutes, or until the chicken reaches an internal temperature of 160°F. Remove from the oven. Let cool for 15 minutes before storing.

STORAGE: Refrigerate the chicken and rice for up to 3 days, or freeze for up to 3 months.

THAWING AND REHEATING: Thaw in the refrigerator overnight. To reheat individual servings, put the chicken and rice in a microwave-safe bowl. Microwave on high power for 30 seconds. Stir the rice. Heat for 30 more seconds, if needed.

Per Serving: Calories: 504; Total fat: 17g; Saturated fat: 8g; Protein: 61g; Total carbs: 24g; Fiber: 3g; Sugar: 3g; Sodium: 783mg

Black Beans and Rice

PREP TIME: 15 MINUTES • COOK TIME: 20 TO 25 MINUTES

Cilantro, sour cream, and avocado are delicious toppings here. The cilantro and sour cream can be prepped in advance. The avocado must be prepped immediately before serving. Whole avocados will keep in the refrigerator for 3 to 5 days. SERVES 4

2 tablespoons extra-virgin olive oil

1 yellow onion, chopped

2 tablespoons minced garlic

2 (15-ounce) cans black beans, drained and rinsed

2 cups vegetable broth

1 teaspoon ground cumin

1 teaspoon sea salt

1 teaspoon dried oregano

1 teaspoon freshly ground black pepper

1 teaspoon dried thyme

2 bay leaves

1 cup salsa verde

2 tablespoons freshly squeezed lime juice

3 cups cooked long-grain white rice

¼ cup full-fat sour cream

¼ cup chopped fresh cilantro

1 ripe avocado, pitted, peeled, and sliced

1. In a large skillet, combine the oil, onion, and garlic. Cook over medium heat, stirring frequently, for 5 to 7 minutes, or until the onion is soft and translucent.

2. Stir in the beans, broth, cumin, salt, oregano, pepper, thyme, bay leaves, and salsa verde. Bring to a boil.

3. Reduce the heat to low. Cover the skillet, and simmer for 15 minutes, stirring occasionally. Remove from the heat. Remove and discard the bay leaves.

4. Stir in the lime juice and rice. Let cool for 10 minutes before storing.

5. Serve the beans and rice with the sour cream, cilantro, and avocado.

STORAGE: Refrigerate the beans and rice for up to 5 days, or freeze for up to 3 months. Divide the sour cream among 4 (2-ounce) serving containers, and refrigerate for up to 1 week. Pat the chopped cilantro dry using a paper towel, and wrap in a fresh paper towel. Put in a storage bag, and squeeze out all the air. Refrigerate for up to 2 weeks.

THAWING AND REHEATING: Thaw in the refrigerator overnight. To heat individual servings, put on a microwave-safe dish, add 1 tablespoon water, and loosely cover with a paper towel. Microwave on high power for 1½ to 2 minutes, stirring every 30 seconds.

Per Serving: Calories: 539; Total fat: 18g; Saturated fat: 4g; Protein: 18g; Total carbs: 79g; Fiber: 18g; Sugar: 6g; Sodium: 953mg

Corn and Salsa Breakfast Burritos

PREP TIME: 10 MINUTES • COOK TIME: 10 MINUTES

Cream-style corn is the secret behind these saucy burritos. Store-bought salsa verde adds flavor without the need to chop peppers, onions, or chilies. Made in minutes, this is an easy breakfast to take on the go. SERVES 4

6 large eggs, beaten

1 (14½-ounce) can cream-style corn

1 cup salsa verde

½ teaspoon sea salt

½ teaspoon freshly ground black pepper

½ cup shredded sharp Cheddar cheese

2 tablespoons salted butter

4 (8-inch) gluten-free flour tortillas

¼ cup chopped fresh cilantro

1 ripe avocado, pitted, peeled, and sliced

1. In a large bowl, stir together the eggs, corn, salsa verde, salt, and pepper until blended.

2. In a large skillet, melt the butter over medium heat.

3. Add the egg mixture, and cook, stirring constantly, for about 5 minutes, or until the eggs are firm. Remove from the heat.

4. Place ¾ cup of the egg mixture across the center of each tortilla. Let cool for 15 minutes.

5. Just before serving, add a sprinkle of cilantro and some avocado.

6. Fold the tortillas burrito-style.

STORAGE: Wrap each burrito tightly in aluminum foil, and put in an airtight container. Keep the avocado and cilantro stored separately. Refrigerate burritos for up to 4 days, or freeze for up to 3 months. Put the cilantro in a storage bag, and squeeze out all the air. Refrigerate for up to 2 weeks.

THAWING AND REHEATING: Thaw in the refrigerator overnight. To reheat individual burritos, put on a microwave-safe plate. Microwave on high power for 1 minute. Heat for 30 seconds to 1 minute more, if needed. Serve sprinkled with cilantro and avocado.

Per Serving: Calories: 550; Total fat: 31g; Saturated fat: 12g; Protein: 20g; Total carbs: 56g; Fiber: 12g; Sugar: 11g; Sodium: 1,420mg

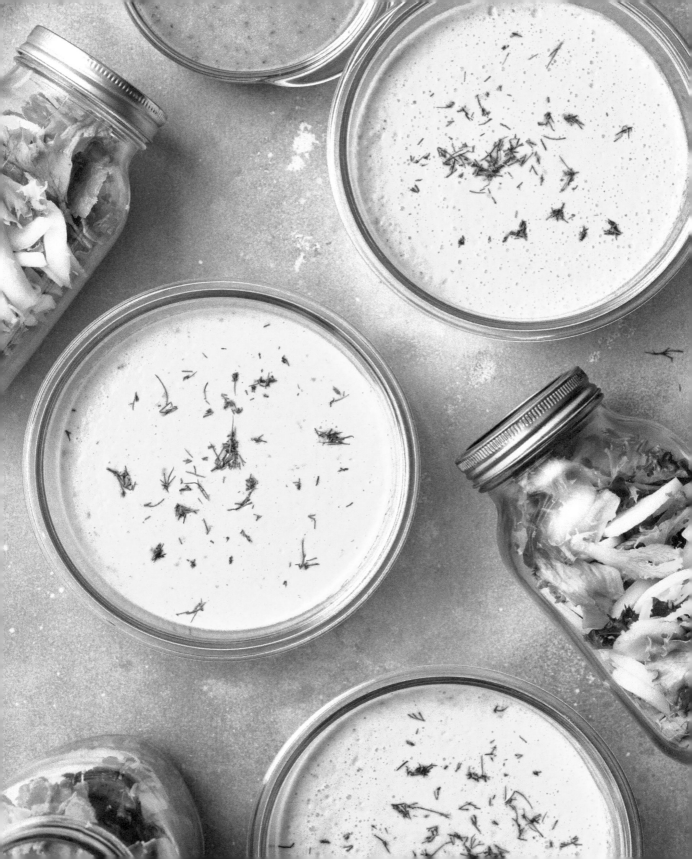

Fixing Up Five: Five-Recipe Meal Preps

'*ve added a recipe to this prep, so expect to spend about 2½ hours in the kitchen. All the recipes are designed to share ingredients and use leftover ingredients as condiments. Pack extras like salsa, sour cream, cheese, and jalapeños in individual serving containers to be used as needed. Our "from scratch" gluten-free fajita seasoning for the Sheet Pan Steak Fajitas (page 57) uses several spices. If you prefer not to purchase them all, substitute 1 (1.12-ounce) packet premade fajita seasoning, but check the ingredient list carefully to ensure it is gluten-free. If you would like to save time prepping vegetables, purchase a jar of minced garlic, usually found in the produce section. Normally, ½ teaspoon jarred minced garlic equals 1 garlic clove, minced.

‹‹ Layered Mixed Greens Salad, page 60; Chilly Cucumber Soup, page 59

SPRING MENU:
Five-Recipe Meal Prep Shopping List

PRODUCE
Avocados (2)
Bell peppers, green, large (2)
Cabbage (1 head)
Carrot (1)
Cilantro (1 bunch)
Cucumbers (2)
Garlic (1 large head)
Lemons (2 or 3)
Limes (2)
Onion, yellow, large (3)
Spring mix (1 [1-pound] package)

DAIRY AND EGGS
Cheese, Cheddar, sharp, shredded
   (1 [1-pound] bag)
Eggs, large (1 dozen)
Milk, 2 percent (1 quart)
Sour cream, full-fat (1 [8-ounce] container)
Yogurt, full-fat, plain (1 [1-pound] container)

MEAT
Bacon (1 [12-ounce] package)
Beef, steak, sirloin, boneless (1 pound)
Crab, imitation, gluten-free (1 [8-ounce]
   package)

CANNED AND BOTTLED
Broth, vegetable (2 [14½-ounce] cans)
Jalapeño peppers, sliced, pickled
   (1 [16-ounce] jar)
Mayonnaise, full-fat (1 [5½-ounce] container)
Water chestnuts, sliced (1 [8-ounce] can)

PANTRY
Crackers, gluten-free (1 package)
Tortillas, flour, 8-inch, gluten-free
   (1 [8-count] package)

CHECK YOUR PANTRY FOR . . .
Balsamic vinegar, black peppercorns, cayenne pepper, chili powder, cornstarch, distilled white vinegar, dried dill, dried mustard, dried parsley, extra-virgin olive oil, garlic powder, gluten-free hot pepper sauce, ground cumin, nonstick cooking spray, onion powder, paprika, sea salt, sugar

Weekly Meal Chart

	BREAKFAST	LUNCH	DINNER
DAY 1	Cheese and Jalapeño Bake	Chilly Cucumber Soup	Crab Coleslaw
DAY 2	Cheese and Jalapeño Bake	Layered Mixed Greens Salad	Chilly Cucumber Soup
DAY 3	Cheese and Jalapeño Bake	Crab Coleslaw	Layered Mixed Greens Salad
DAY 4	Cheese and Jalapeño Bake	Layered Mixed Greens Salad	Chilly Cucumber Soup
DAY 5	Cheese and Jalapeño Bake	Crab Coleslaw	Sheet Pan Steak Fajitas
DAY 6		Chilly Cucumber Soup	Sheet Pan Steak Fajitas

STEP-BY-STEP PREP

1. Prep the vegetables for the week:

- ☐ *Peel and thinly slice 2 cucumbers.*

- ☐ *Chop enough cilantro to measure ½ cup.*

- ☐ *Shred enough cabbage to measure 3 cups.*

- ☐ *Thinly slice 1 yellow onion. Chop 1 or 2 onions until you have 2¼ cups. Divide the chopped onion into 2 (1-cup) and 1 (¼-cup) portions.*

- ☐ *Peel and shred 1 carrot.*

- ☐ *Juice enough lemons to measure 2 tablespoons juice.*

- ☐ *Juice enough limes to measure 2 tablespoons juice.*

- ☐ *Mince enough garlic to measure 3 tablespoons.*

☐ *Seed and slice 1 green bell pepper, and seed and chop enough of the other green bell pepper to measure 1 cup.*

2. Boil the eggs. Put 4 eggs in a medium saucepan, and add enough water to cover. Bring to a rolling boil over high heat. Reduce the heat to medium-low. Cover the pan, and cook for 5 minutes. Remove from the heat. Let sit for 5 minutes. Rinse the eggs under cold water, peel, and slice. Rinse the saucepan.

3. Cook the bacon. In a large skillet, cook 12 bacon slices (or 8 slices if you are omitting the bacon from the Cheese and Jalapeño Bake) over medium heat, turning every 2 to 3 minutes, for 7 to 10 minutes, or until they reach your desired crispness. Remove from the heat. Transfer to paper towels to drain and cool. Crumble the bacon.

4. Prepare the Cheese and Jalapeño Bake (page 56) as directed. Let cool for 20 minutes. Put in an airtight container, or tightly wrap with aluminum foil. Refrigerate for up to 5 days, or freeze for up to 2 months. In each of 4 (2-ounce) containers, combine 1 tablespoon sour cream and 1 tablespoon chopped cilantro, and refrigerate

for up to 7 days. The avocado must be prepped the day of serving.

5. Prepare the Sheet Pan Steak Fajitas (page 57) as directed. Let cool for 15 minutes. Put the meat mixture in an airtight container, and refrigerate for up to 4 days, or freeze for up to 3 months. Unopened packaged tortillas are shelf stable for 1 week, can be refrigerated for 1 month, and can be frozen for 6 months. Divide ½ cup Cheddar cheese among 4 (2-ounce) containers. Refrigerate for up to 2 weeks. In each of 4 (4-ounce) containers, combine 1 tablespoon sour cream, 1 tablespoon chopped cilantro, and 2 tablespoons jalapeños (if using), and refrigerate for up to 7 days. The avocado must be prepped the day of serving.

6. Prepare the Chilly Cucumber Soup (page 59) as directed. Put in an airtight container, and refrigerate for up to 5 days. Serve chilled. This soup should not be frozen.

7. Prepare the Layered Mixed Greens Salad (page 60) as directed. Put the salad in an airtight container, and refrigerate for up to 4 days. Divide the dressing among 4 (2-ounce) containers,

and refrigerate for up to 5 days.
The salad and dressing cannot
be frozen.

8. Prepare the Crab Coleslaw
   (page 61) as directed. Put the
   coleslaw in an airtight container,
   and refrigerate for up to 5 days.
   Because of the mayonnaise-based
   dressing, this should not be frozen.

Cheese and Jalapeño Bake

PREP TIME: 10 MINUTES • COOK TIME: 30 MINUTES

Jalapeños are the star of this dish, adding heat and a touch of South-western flavor to the fluffy eggs. Adjust the amount and type of hot sauce for your personal preference. **SERVES 5**

Nonstick cooking spray, for coating the baking dish

8 large eggs, beaten

1¾ cups 2 percent milk

2 cups shredded sharp Cheddar cheese

1 teaspoon gluten-free hot pepper sauce

1 teaspoon sea salt

½ teaspoon freshly ground black pepper

1 cup pickled jalapeño pepper slices, chopped

4 bacon slices, cooked, drained, and crumbled (optional)

¼ cup full-fat sour cream

¼ cup chopped fresh cilantro

1 ripe avocado, pitted, peeled, and sliced

1. Preheat the oven to 350°F. Coat a 9-by-9-inch baking dish with cooking spray.

2. In a large bowl, whisk together the eggs, milk, cheese, hot pepper sauce, salt, pepper, jalapeños, and bacon (if using) until blended.

3. Pour the egg mixture into the prepared baking dish.

4. Transfer the baking dish to the oven, and bake for 25 to 30 minutes, or until a knife inserted into the center comes out clean. Remove from the oven. Let cool for 20 minutes.

5. Serve the baked eggs with the sour cream, cilantro, and avocado.

STORAGE: Put in an airtight container, or tightly wrap with aluminum foil. Refrigerate for up to 5 days, or freeze for up to 2 months. In each of 4 (2-ounce) storage containers, combine 1 tablespoon sour cream and 1 tablespoon chopped cilantro, and refrigerate for up to 7 days. The avocado must be prepped the day of serving.

THAWING AND REHEATING: Thaw in the refrigerator overnight. To reheat individual servings, loosely wrap with a damp paper towel. Microwave on 50 percent power for 45 seconds. Heat for 15 to 30 more seconds, if needed.

VARIATION TIP: Add 1 pound cooked crumbled hot pork sausage to the egg mixture before baking.

Per Serving: Calories: 445; Total fat: 33g; Saturated fat: 15g; Protein: 26g; Total carbs: 13g; Fiber: 3g; Sugar: 8g; Sodium: 843mg

Sheet Pan Steak Fajitas

PREP TIME: 20 MINUTES • COOK TIME: 15 MINUTES

The fajita seasoning can be made in advance and doubled or tripled. Store it in an airtight container for up to 6 months. Increase the cayenne pepper to 1 teaspoon for more heat. SERVES 4

For the fajita seasoning mix

1 tablespoon cornstarch

2 teaspoons chili powder

1 teaspoon sea salt

1 teaspoon paprika

1 teaspoon sugar

1 teaspoon onion powder

1 teaspoon garlic powder

1 teaspoon ground cumin

½ teaspoon cayenne pepper

For the fajitas

Nonstick cooking spray, for coating the sheet pan

1 large yellow onion, thinly sliced

1 large green bell pepper, sliced

1 pound boneless sirloin steak, cut into 1-inch-thick slices

¼ cup extra-virgin olive oil

2 tablespoons freshly squeezed lime juice

½ cup shredded sharp Cheddar cheese

¼ cup full-fat sour cream

¼ cup chopped fresh cilantro

½ cup pickled jalapeño pepper slices (optional)

To make the fajita seasoning mix

1. In a medium bowl, stir together the cornstarch, chili powder, salt, paprika, sugar, onion powder, garlic powder, ground cumin, and cayenne until blended.

To make the fajitas

2. Preheat the oven to 400°F. Coat a large sheet pan with cooking spray.

3. In a large bowl, combine the fajita seasoning mix, onion, bell pepper, and steak.

4. Pour the oil over everything, and using your clean hands, toss to coat.

5. Spread the mixture evenly across the prepared sheet pan.

6. Transfer the sheet pan to the oven, and bake, stirring every 5 minutes, for 10 to 12 minutes, or until the steak reaches an internal temperature of 140°F. Remove from the oven.

7. Sprinkle the fajita mixture with the lime juice. Let cool for 15 minutes.

8. Divide the cheese among 4 (2-ounce) containers.

9. In each of 4 (4-ounce) containers, combine 1 tablespoon of sour cream, 1 tablespoon of cilantro, and 2 tablespoons of jalapeño pepper slices.

10. Serve the fajita mixture with the cheese, sour cream mixture, tortillas, and avocado.

CONTINUED ⟶

8 (8-inch) gluten-free flour tortillas

1 ripe avocado, pitted, peeled, and sliced

STORAGE: Refrigerate the meat mixture in an airtight container for up to 4 days, or freeze for up to 3 months. Unopened packaged tortillas are shelf stable for 1 week, can be refrigerated for 1 month, and can be frozen for 6 months. Refrigerate the sour cream mixture for up to 7 days. Refrigerate the cheese for up to 2 weeks. The avocado must be prepped the day of serving.

THAWING AND REHEATING: Thaw the meat mixture in the refrigerator overnight. To reheat individual servings, put on a microwave-safe dish, and cover with a damp paper towel. Microwave on 50 percent power for 1 minute. Stir and heat for 30 more seconds, if needed. Place the meat mixture on the tortilla, and add the toppings.

SUBSTITUTION TIP: Swap in 1 pound boneless, skinless chicken breasts or pork roast strips for the steak. Replace the gluten-free flour tortillas with corn tortillas.

Per Serving: Calories: 856; Total fat: 50g; Saturated fat: 17g; Protein: 36g; Total carbs: 70g; Fiber: 17g; Sugar: 12g; Sodium: 1,540mg

Chilly Cucumber Soup

PREP TIME: 15 MINUTES • COOK TIME: 15 MINUTES

We may crave hot, hearty soups in winter, but this cool, creamy soup, with a hint of dill, garlic, and onion, makes for a tempting light lunch in spring and summer. Look for firm, dark green cucumbers with no soft spots. Soft softs indicate that a cucumber is beginning to rot. **SERVES 4**

2 cucumbers, peeled and thinly sliced

1 teaspoon sea salt

2 cups vegetable broth

¼ cup chopped yellow onion

1 tablespoon minced garlic

2 cups full-fat plain yogurt

½ cup 2 percent milk

1 teaspoon dried dill

½ teaspoon freshly ground black pepper

1. Put the cucumber slices on a paper towel. Pat dry using more paper towel, and sprinkle with the salt. Let sit for 5 minutes to remove excess moisture. Pat the cucumbers dry again.

2. In a medium saucepan, combine the broth, cucumbers, onion, and garlic. Bring to a boil over medium heat. Cook for 15 minutes, or until the cucumbers are soft and easily pierced with a fork. Remove from the heat. Let cool for 15 minutes. Transfer to a blender.

3. Add the yogurt, milk, dill, and pepper. Blend for 10 to 15 seconds, or until pureed.

STORAGE: Put in an airtight container. Refrigerate for up to 5 days. Serve chilled. This soup should not be frozen because the texture and consistency will change if frozen.

SUBSTITUTION TIP: Swap out the dried dill and vegetable broth for 2 tablespoons chopped fresh dill and 3 cups chicken broth.

Per Serving: Calories: 116; Total fat: 5g; Saturated fat: 3g; Protein: 6g; Total carbs: 12g; Fiber: 1g; Sugar: 10g; Sodium: 656mg

Layered Mixed Greens Salad

PREP TIME: 20 MINUTES

A tangy dressing gives this classic salad new life. When purchasing mixed greens, look for colorful leaves with no wilting or brown or yellow spots. Mixed greens should be stored unwashed in the refrigerator before use. **SERVES 4**

For the salad

1 (16-ounce) package
   spring mix
8 bacon slices, cooked,
   drained, and crumbled
1 cup chopped onion
4 large hard-boiled eggs,
   peeled and sliced
1 (8-ounce) can sliced water
   chestnuts, drained
1 cup shredded sharp
   Cheddar cheese

For the dressing

2 tablespoons minced garlic
2 tablespoons sugar
1½ teaspoons sea salt
1 teaspoon dried parsley
½ teaspoon freshly ground
   black pepper
½ teaspoon dried mustard
¼ cup full-fat sour cream
1 cup extra-virgin olive oil
½ cup balsamic vinegar

To make the salad

1. To prepare individual salads, in each of 4 (1-pint) Mason jars, put 1 cup of mixed greens.

2. Divide the bacon, onion, eggs, water chestnuts, and Cheddar cheese among the salads. To make 1 large salad, in a large airtight container, layer the salad ingredients as listed.

To make the dressing

3. In a small bowl, whisk together the garlic, sugar, salt, parsley, pepper, and mustard to blend.

4. Add the sour cream, and whisk until blended.

5. Whisk in the oil and vinegar. Whisk or shake well before using.

STORAGE: Refrigerate the salad in an airtight container for up to 4 days. Divide the dressing among 4 (2-ounce) containers, and refrigerate for up to 5 days. The salad and dressing cannot be frozen. The greens will become mushy, the eggs will become rubbery, and the texture and consistency of the dressing will change if frozen.

INGREDIENT TIP: Unpeeled hard-boiled eggs can be prepared up to 7 days in advance and kept refrigerated in an airtight container.

Per Serving: Calories: 1,003; Total fat: 80g; Saturated fat: 19g; Protein: 24g; Total carbs: 49g; Fiber: 2g; Sugar: 15g; Sodium: 1,403mg

Crab Coleslaw

PREP TIME: 15 MINUTES

Imitation crab meat sometimes uses gluten as a binder. Check the ingredients on the package to be sure your crab is gluten-free. Real crab can be substituted for the imitation crab. SERVES 4

For the dressing

½ cup full-fat mayonnaise

2 tablespoons sugar

2 tablespoons freshly squeezed lemon juice

1 tablespoon distilled white vinegar

1 teaspoon sea salt

½ teaspoon freshly ground black pepper

For the coleslaw

1 (8-ounce) package gluten-free imitation crab, chopped (see ingredient tip)

3 cups shredded cabbage

1 carrot, shredded

1 cup chopped yellow onion

1 cup chopped green bell pepper

½ cup pickled jalapeño pepper slices (optional)

Gluten-free crackers, for serving

To make the dressing

1. In a small bowl, whisk together the mayonnaise, sugar, lemon juice, vinegar, salt, and pepper until blended and smooth.

To make the coleslaw

2. In a large bowl, gently stir together the crab, cabbage, carrot, onion, bell pepper, and jalapeños (if using).

3. Add the dressing, and gently stir to coat and combine.

STORAGE: Put in an airtight container. Refrigerate for up to 5 days. Because of the mayonnaise-based dressing, this slaw does not freeze well.

INGREDIENT TIP: Imitation crab often contains wheat binders, so not all brands are gluten-free. Check the ingredients before purchasing.

Per Serving: Calories: 318; Total fat: 21g; Saturated fat: 3g; Protein: 6g; Total carbs: 27g; Fiber: 3g; Sugar: 16g; Sodium: 987mg

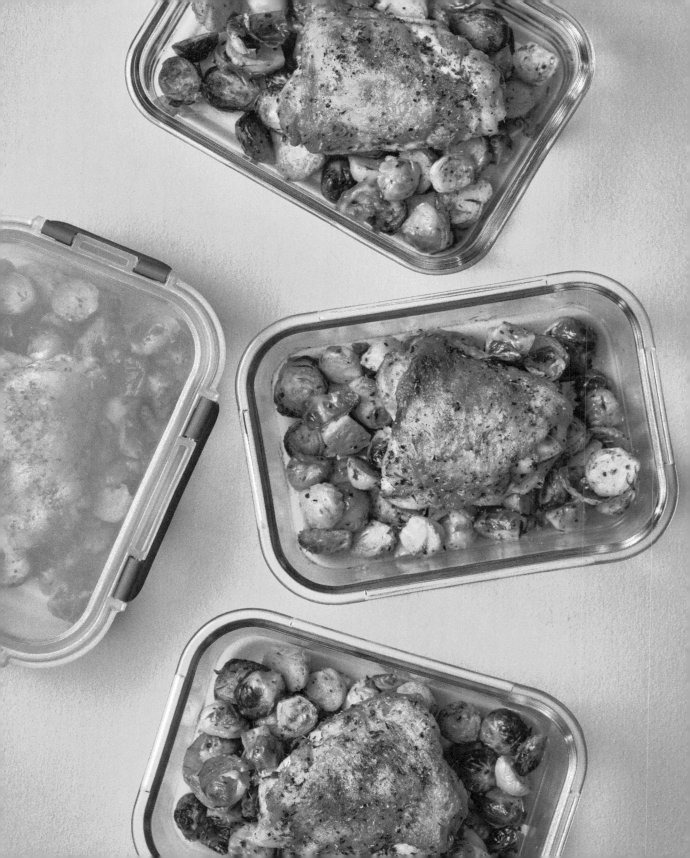

SUMMER MENU:
Five-Recipe Meal Prep

Summer brings new twists on old favorites. I've taken a traditional rice dish and replaced the rice with broccoli. A chicken and pasta dish gets remade with quinoa. The salad can be made in minutes, thanks to using a bag of packaged spring mix as a base. Even the gumbo is streamlined to be ready in about 30 minutes of cooking time. Try the chocolate smoothie for breakfast, as a snack, or as dessert. It's thick and rich enough to have the mouthfeel of a milk shake but has no added sugar. If you're not a chocolate fan, replace the smoothie with the Very Berry Smoothie (page 30), the Peach and Pineapple Smoothie (page 118), or any of the breakfasts in chapter 5. Check your pantry, and replace the broccoli rice with your rice of choice, quinoa, or millet. When shopping, choose your favorite flavor of goat cheese to accompany the salad.

‹‹ Herbed Sheet Pan Chicken with Brussels Sprouts, page 77

SUMMER MENU:
Five-Recipe Meal Prep Shopping List

PRODUCE
Bananas, large (4)
Bell peppers, green (3)
Broccoli (1 head)
Celery (1 bunch)
Garlic (2 heads)
Lemons (2 or 3)
Mushrooms (1 [8-ounce] container)
Onions, yellow (4)
Spring mix (1 [1-pound] package)
Tomatoes, cherry (1 [8-ounce] package)

DAIRY AND EGGS
Cheese, Cheddar, sharp, shredded
 (1 [8-ounce] bag)
Cheese, goat, crumbled (1 [8-ounce]
 package)
Milk, 2 percent (1 pint)

MEAT
Beef, ground, 80/20 (1 pound)
Chicken, breasts, boneless, skinless
 (1½ pounds)

FROZEN FOOD
Peas and carrots (1 [10-ounce] package)
Shrimp, medium, peeled, deveined, tails off
 (1 pound)

CANNED AND BOTTLED
Banana peppers, mild, sliced
 (1 [15-ounce] jar)
Broth, beef (1 [14½-ounce] can)
Broth, chicken (1 [32-ounce] container)
Olives, black, sliced (2 [7-ounce] cans)
Peanut butter, smooth (1 [1-pound] jar)
Tomatoes, crushed (1 [28-ounce] can)
Tomatoes, diced (1 [14½-ounce] can)

PANTRY
Quinoa (1 [12-ounce] package)
Rice, long-grain, white (1 [8-ounce]
 package)

CHECK YOUR PANTRY FOR . . .
Black peppercorns, canola oil,
chili powder, cocoa powder, cornstarch, dried oregano, dried thyme,
extra-virgin olive oil, gluten-free hot
pepper sauce, Italian seasoning, sea
salt, vanilla extract

Weekly Meal Chart

	BREAKFAST	LUNCH	DINNER
DAY 1	Chocolate–Peanut Butter Smoothie	Layered Greek Salad	Lemon Chicken and Quinoa
DAY 2	Chocolate–Peanut Butter Smoothie	Snappy Shrimp Gumbo	Layered Greek Salad
DAY 3		Layered Greek Salad	Lemon Chicken and Quinoa
DAY 4	Chocolate–Peanut Butter Smoothie	Layered Greek Salad	Beefy Spanish Broccoli "Rice"
DAY 5	Chocolate–Peanut Butter Smoothie	Beefy Spanish Broccoli "Rice"	Snappy Shrimp Gumbo
DAY 6		Beefy Spanish Broccoli "Rice"	Lemon Chicken and Quinoa

STEP-BY-STEP PREP

1. Peel and slice 4 bananas, and put in an airtight container. Freeze.

2. Cook the quinoa. Rinse 1 cup quinoa in a strainer. In a large saucepan, combine 1¾ cups water and the quinoa. Bring to a boil over high heat. Stir. Reduce the heat to low, cover the pan, and simmer for 18 to 20 minutes. Remove from the heat. Let rest for 5 minutes before using.

3. While the quinoa cooks, prep the vegetables for the week:

   ☐ *Dice enough yellow onion to measure 1 cup. Chop enough of the remaining onions until you have 3 (1-cup) portions.*

   ☐ *Seed and dice enough green bell pepper to measure 1 cup. Seed and chop enough of the remaining peppers until you have 2 (1-cup) portions.*

☐ *Dice enough celery to measure ½ cup.*

☐ *Slice 8 ounces mushrooms.*

☐ *Juice 2 or 3 lemons to measure ¼ cup juice.*

☐ *Mince enough garlic to measure ¼ cup plus 1 teaspoon.*

☐ *Rice 1 head broccoli. Remove the florets from the stalk. Chop the florets into large pieces. Using the largest holes on a cheese grater or box grater, grate the broccoli florets until they resemble grains of rice. Or use a blender, and pulse for 5 to 10 seconds, or until the broccoli resembles rice.*

4. Cook the rice. Rinse out the saucepan, and put 1⅓ cups water and ⅔ cup long-grain white rice in it. Bring to a boil over high heat. Reduce the heat to low. Cover the pan, and simmer for 15 minutes, or until tender. Remove from the heat. Let rest for 10 minutes.

5. Cook the ground beef. In a large skillet, cook 1 pound ground beef over medium heat, breaking up the beef, for 5 to 7 minutes, or until no pink remains. Remove from the heat. Drain. Wash the skillet.

6. Cook the broccoli. In the same skillet, combine 2 tablespoons olive oil and 3 cups riced broccoli. Cook over medium heat, stirring often, for 5 minutes, or until tender and fluffy. Remove from the heat. Let cool. If not using immediately, put in an airtight container, refrigerate for up to 1 week, or freeze for up to 6 months.

7. Prepare the Beefy Spanish Broccoli "Rice" (page 68) as directed. Let cool for 15 minutes. Put in an airtight container. Refrigerate for up to 5 days, or freeze for up to 3 months.

8. Prepare the Snappy Shrimp Gumbo (page 69) as directed. Let cool for 15 minutes. Put in an airtight container, and refrigerate for up to 3 days, or freeze for up to 3 months.

9. Prepare the Lemon Chicken and Quinoa (page 70) as directed. Let cool for 15 minutes. Put in an airtight container. Refrigerate for up to 3 days, or freeze for up to 3 months.

10. Prepare the Layered Greek Salad (page 71) as directed. Seal the Mason jars. Put 1 tablespoon salad dressing in each of 4 (1-ounce) containers. Refrigerate the salad

for up to 5 days and the dressing
for up to 1 week.

11. Remove the bananas from the
freezer. Prepare the Chocolate–
Peanut Butter Smoothie (page 72)
as directed. Seal the jars, and
refrigerate for up to 5 days, or
freeze for up to 3 months.

Beefy Spanish Broccoli "Rice"

PREP TIME: 15 MINUTES • COOK TIME: 35 MINUTES

The Spaniards discovered rice in Asia and introduced it to Mexico. The result was a traditional dish named "Spanish rice." I've taken out the white rice and replaced it with broccoli. **SERVES 4**

¼ cup canola oil

1 cup chopped yellow onion

1 cup chopped green bell pepper

1 pound 80/20 ground beef, cooked, crumbled, and drained

1 (28-ounce) can crushed tomatoes

1 (14½-ounce) can beef broth

¾ cup sliced black olives

1 teaspoon sea salt

½ teaspoon freshly ground black pepper

2 tablespoons chili powder

3 cups cooked "riced" broccoli

1 cup shredded sharp Cheddar cheese

1. In a large skillet, combine the oil, onion, and bell pepper. Cook over medium heat, stirring often, for 7 to 10 minutes, or until the onion is tender and translucent.

2. Add the beef, tomatoes, broth, olives, salt, and pepper. Bring to a boil.

3. Reduce the heat to low. Cover the skillet, and simmer, stirring occasionally, for 20 minutes, or until the mixture has slightly thickened. Remove from the heat.

4. Stir in the chili powder and broccoli. Evenly sprinkle the cheese on top. Let cool for 15 minutes.

STORAGE: Put in an airtight container. Refrigerate for up to 5 days, or freeze for up to 3 months.

THAWING AND REHEATING: Thaw in the refrigerator overnight. To reheat individual servings, put in a microwave-safe bowl, and loosely cover with a paper towel. Microwave on 50 percent power for 1 minute. Stir and heat for 30 more seconds.

SUBSTITUTION TIP: Swap in 1 pound cooked crumbled Italian sausage for the ground beef. For additional flavor, add 1 (4½-ounce) can green chilies, drained and diced.

Per Serving: Calories: 625; Total fat: 50g; Saturated fat: 16g; Protein: 30g; Total carbs: 17g; Fiber: 8g; Sugar: 8g; Sodium: 1,179mg

Snappy Shrimp Gumbo

PREP TIME: 20 MINUTES • COOK TIME: 30 MINUTES

Long, slow-cooked gumbos are a mainstay in Creole and Cajun cultures. They're delicious—but require a complicated cooking process. This simple recipe features the ingredients found in the dish but reduces the cooking time. SERVES 4

2 tablespoons extra-virgin
   olive oil

1 cup chopped yellow onion

1 cup chopped green
   bell pepper

½ cup diced celery

2 tablespoons minced garlic

2 cups chicken broth

1 (14½-ounce) can diced
   tomatoes

1 teaspoon dried oregano

1 teaspoon dried thyme

1 teaspoon chili powder

1 teaspoon sea salt

½ teaspoon freshly ground
   black pepper

1 tablespoon gluten-free hot
   pepper sauce

1 pound frozen medium
   shrimp, peeled, deveined,
   tails removed, at room
   temperature for 15 minutes
   before using

2 cups cooked long-grain
   white rice

1. In a large skillet, combine the oil, onion, bell pepper, celery, and garlic. Cook over medium heat, stirring often, for 5 to 7 minutes, or until the onion is soft and opaque.

2. Stir in the broth and tomatoes with their juices.

3. In a small bowl, stir together the oregano, thyme, chili powder, salt, and pepper. Stir into the skillet.

4. Add the hot sauce, and bring the mixture to a boil.

5. Reduce the heat to low. Cover the skillet, and simmer, stirring occasionally, for 15 minutes, or until the mixture has slightly thickened.

6. Stir in the shrimp, and cook, stirring often, for 3 to 4 minutes, or until the shrimp are soft and white. Remove from the heat.

7. Stir in the rice. Let cool for 15 minutes.

STORAGE: Put in an airtight container. Refrigerate for up to 3 days, or freeze for up to 3 months.

THAWING AND REHEATING: Thaw in the refrigerator overnight. To reheat individual servings, put in a microwave-safe dish, and cover with a paper towel. Microwave on high power for 30 seconds. Stir and heat for 30 more seconds. Stir before serving.

- -

Per Serving: Calories: 294; Total fat: 9g; Saturated fat: 1g; Protein: 20g; Total carbs: 35g; Fiber: 4g; Sugar: 6g; Sodium: 1,321mg

Lemon Chicken and Quinoa

PREP TIME: 15 MINUTES • COOK TIME: 20 MINUTES

Tender chunks of chicken mix with peas and carrots in a lemony sauce in this quick-to-prepare dish, while quinoa stands in for rice to provide a nutty flavor. Use leftover sliced banana peppers to garnish, if desired. SERVES 4

¼ cup canola oil

1½ pounds boneless, skinless chicken breasts, diced

1 cup chopped yellow onion

2 tablespoons minced garlic

1 tablespoon cornstarch

2 cups chicken broth

1 teaspoon Italian seasoning

½ teaspoon sea salt

3 tablespoons freshly squeezed lemon juice

1 (10-ounce) package frozen peas and carrots

3 cups cooked quinoa

½ cup sliced mild banana peppers (optional)

1. In a large skillet, combine the oil and chicken. Cook over medium heat, stirring often, for 5 to 7 minutes, or until the chicken is no longer pink.

2. Add the onion and garlic. Cook for 5 minutes, or until the onion is tender.

3. To make a slurry, in a small bowl, whisk together the cornstarch and broth until dissolved.

4. Whisk the Italian seasoning, salt, and lemon juice into the slurry.

5. Add the slurry to the chicken mixture.

6. Stir in the peas and carrots. Cook, stirring often, for about 7 minutes, or until the mixture thickens and the peas and carrots are soft. Remove from the heat.

7. Stir in the quinoa and banana peppers (if using). Let cool for 15 minutes.

STORAGE: Put in an airtight container. Refrigerate for up to 3 days, or freeze for up to 3 months.

THAWING AND REHEATING: Thaw in the refrigerator overnight. To reheat individual servings, put in a microwave-safe container. Microwave on high power for 30 seconds. Stir and heat for 30 more seconds. Stir before serving.

- -

Per Serving: Calories: 542; Total fat: 19g; Saturated fat: 2g; Protein: 47g; Total carbs: 45g; Fiber: 7g; Sugar: 3g; Sodium: 446mg

Layered Greek Salad

PREP TIME: 20 MINUTES

From sliced ripe olives, banana peppers, and crumbled goat cheese, the flavors of the Mediterranean are highlighted in this classic salad. Serve with a glass of wine, and feel as if you're spending the day in Greece. SERVES 4

For the salad

1 (1-pound) package spring mix

1 cup diced yellow onion

1 cup diced green bell pepper

1 (8-ounce) container mushrooms, sliced

1 cup sliced black olives

1 cup sliced mild banana peppers

1 (8-ounce) package cherry tomatoes

1 (8-ounce) package crumbled goat cheese

For the Greek dressing

¼ cup extra-virgin olive oil

1 tablespoon freshly squeezed lemon juice

2 teaspoons dried oregano

1 teaspoon minced garlic

½ teaspoon freshly ground black pepper

To make the salad

1. To prepare individual salads, in each of 4 (1-pint) Mason jars, put 1 cup of spring mix.

2. Top each salad with the following, in the order listed: ¼ cup of onion, ¼ cup of bell pepper, ¼ cup of mushrooms, ¼ cup of olives, ¼ cup of banana peppers, ¼ cup of cherry tomatoes, and ¼ cup of goat cheese. To prepare 1 large salad, in a large bowl or on a serving platter, layer the ingredients in the order listed.

To make the Greek dressing

3. In a large measuring cup, whisk together the oil, lemon juice, oregano, garlic, and pepper until blended. Immediately before serving, pour over the salad, and toss to coat.

STORAGE: Put 1 tablespoon of salad dressing in each of 4 (1-ounce) containers. Refrigerate the salad for up to 5 days and the dressing for up to 1 week. The salad should not be frozen, because the greens will become mushy.

VARIATION TIP: Top each salad with ¼ to ½ cup thinly sliced grilled steak or diced grilled chicken.

Per Serving: Calories: 287; Total fat: 22g; Saturated fat: 6g; Protein: 9g; Total carbs: 17g; Fiber: 6g; Sugar: 7g; Sodium: 363mg

Chocolate-Peanut Butter Smoothie

PREP TIME: 10 MINUTES

This smooth, creamy smoothie gets its natural sweetness from banana. Reminiscent of a banana split, except packed with protein, fiber, and magnesium, you'll never notice this frosty drink doesn't include sugar. SERVES 4

4 large bananas, peeled, sliced, and frozen

½ cup smooth peanut butter

1½ cups 2 percent milk

2 tablespoons unsweetened cocoa powder

1 teaspoon vanilla extract

1. In a high-speed blender, combine the bananas, peanut butter, and milk. Pulse for 20 seconds.

2. Add the cocoa powder and vanilla. Pulse for 10 seconds, or until blended and smooth.

3. To prepare individual servings, pour the smoothie into 4 (8-ounce) Mason jars. Seal the jars.

STORAGE: Refrigerate for up to 5 days, or freeze for up to 3 months.

THAWING AND REHEATING: Thaw in the refrigerator overnight. Stir before serving.

VARIATION TIP:

CHOCOLATE-STRAWBERRY SMOOTHIE: Replace the peanut butter with 1 (10-ounce) package frozen strawberries.

CHOCOLATE CHIP PROTEIN SMOOTHIE: Replace the peanut butter with 2 scoops vanilla or chocolate protein powder. Stir in ¼ cup mini semisweet chocolate chips.

CHOCOLATE-MINT SMOOTHIE: Replace the peanut butter with 1 teaspoon mint extract.

CHOCOLATE DESSERT SMOOTHIE: Replace the milk with 2 cups vanilla ice cream. For an alcoholic dessert version, replace the peanut butter with 2 tablespoons Kahlúa and the milk with 2 cups vanilla ice cream.

- -

Per Serving: Calories: 369; Total fat: 19g; Saturated fat: 5g; Protein: 12g; Total carbs: 44g; Fiber: 6g; Sugar: 25g; Sodium: 50mg

FALL MENU:
Five-Recipe Meal Prep

This fall menu will warm you up with classic comfort foods like potato soup loaded with cheese and muffins filled with that perennial favorite fall flavor—pumpkin spice. Sheet pans work their magic to prepare herbed chicken and crispy-on-the-outside Brussels sprouts. And whip out that skillet because we'll be simmering a simple spaghetti dish right on the stovetop. We'll even visit New Orleans without ever leaving home with spicy black-eyed peas served with lentils. Don't forget to be a pantry shopper before your trip to the store. You'll have several leftover eggs this week. Use them to prepare Egg Salad Sandwiches (page 93) or a batch of Three-Cheese Omelets with Bacon (page 155). Leftover chicken broth and canned pumpkin can be frozen in airtight containers and used later in Oatmeal "Meatballs" with Pumpkin Sauce (page 145).

FALL MENU:
Five-Recipe Meal Prep Shopping List

PRODUCE
Bell peppers, green (2)
Brussels sprouts (2 pounds)
Celery (1 bunch)
Garlic (1 head)
Onions, yellow (3)
Potatoes, Russet (4)

DAIRY AND EGGS
**Cheese, Cheddar, sharp, shredded
  (1 [8-ounce] bag)**
Eggs, large (1 half dozen)
Milk, 2 percent (1 pint)

MEAT
Bacon (1 [12-ounce] package)
Beef, ground 80/20 (1 pound)
Chicken, bone-in thighs (4 [8-ounce])

CANNED AND BOTTLED
Black-eyed peas (1 [15½-ounce] can)
Broth, beef (1 [32-ounce] container)
Broth, chicken (1 [32-ounce] container)
Pumpkin (1 [15-ounce] can)
Tomatoes, diced (1 [28-ounce] can)
Tomato sauce (1 [8-ounce] can)

PANTRY
**All-purpose gluten-free one-to-one baking
  flour (1 [1-pound] package)**
Lentils, brown (1 [8-ounce] package)
**Spaghetti, gluten-free (1 [12-ounce]
  package)**
Sugar, granulated white (1 [1-pound] bag)

CHECK YOUR PANTRY FOR . . .
Baking soda, black peppercorns,
canola oil, cayenne pepper, chili
powder, curry powder, dried
basil, dried mustard, dried thyme,
extra-virgin olive oil, ground cinnamon, ground cumin, ground nutmeg,
Italian seasoning, nonstick cooking
spray, onion powder, paprika, sea salt

Weekly Meal Chart

	BREAKFAST	LUNCH	DINNER
DAY 1	Pumpkin Spice Muffins	Cheesy Potato Soup	Herbed Sheet Pan Chicken with Brussels Sprouts
DAY 2	Pumpkin Spice Muffins	Skillet Spaghetti	Creole Black-Eyed Peas with Lentils
DAY 3	Pumpkin Spice Muffins	Cheesy Potato Soup	Herbed Sheet Pan Chicken with Brussels Sprouts
DAY 4	Pumpkin Spice Muffins	Creole Black-Eyed Peas with Lentils	Skillet Spaghetti
DAY 5	Pumpkin Spice Muffins	Herbed Sheet Pan Chicken with Brussels Sprouts	Cheesy Potato Soup
DAY 6	Pumpkin Spice Muffins	Skillet Spaghetti	Creole Black-Eyed Peas with Lentils

STEP-BY-STEP PREP

1. Prep the vegetables for the week:

   ☐ *Trim and halve 2 pounds Brussels sprouts.*

   ☐ *Chop 3 yellow onions, and divide into 3 (1-cup) portions.*

   ☐ *Seed and chop 2 green bell peppers, and divide into 2 (1-cup) portions.*

   ☐ *Chop enough celery to measure ½ cup.*

   ☐ *Dice enough potatoes to measure 4 cups.*

   ☐ *Mince enough garlic to measure 3 tablespoons.*

2. Cook the lentils. Rinse 1¼ cups brown lentils in a strainer. In a

large saucepan, combine 3¾ cups water and the lentils. Bring to a boil over high heat. Reduce the heat to low. Stir, cover the pan, and simmer for 18 to 20 minutes, or until tender. Remove from the heat. Let sit for 5 minutes before using. Drain any excess water from the lentils.

3. Cook the bacon. In a large skillet, cook 12 bacon slices (or just 8 if omitting the bacon from the Cheesy Potato Soup) over medium heat, turning every 2 to 3 minutes, for 7 to 10 minutes, or until they reach your desired crispness. Remove from the heat. Transfer to paper towels to drain and cool. Crumble the bacon. Rinse the skillet.

4. Cook the ground beef. In the same skillet, cook 1 pound ground beef over medium heat for 7 to 10 minutes, or until browned and no pink remains. Drain.

5. Prepare the Herbed Sheet Pan Chicken with Brussels Sprouts (page 77) as directed. Let cool for 15 minutes. Put in an airtight container. Refrigerate for up to 4 days, or freeze for up to 3 months.

6. Prepare the Cheesy Potato Soup (page 78) as directed. Let cool for 15 to 20 minutes. Put in an airtight container. Refrigerate for up to 4 days, or freeze for up to 3 months. Put 1 crumbled bacon slice in each of 4 (1-ounce) containers (if using), and refrigerate for up to 5 days, or freeze for up to 1 month.

7. Prepare the Skillet Spaghetti (page 79) as directed. Let cool for 15 minutes. Put in an airtight container, making sure the pasta is covered with sauce. Refrigerate for up to 5 days, or freeze for up to 3 months.

8. Prepare the Creole Black-Eyed Peas with Lentils (page 80) as directed. Let cool for 15 to 20 minutes. Put in an airtight container. Refrigerate for up to 5 days, or freeze for up to 3 months.

9. Prepare the Pumpkin Spice Muffins (page 81) as directed. Let cool for 15 to 20 minutes. Put in an airtight container. Store at room temperature for up to 3 days, refrigerate for up to 7 days, or freeze for up to 3 months.

Herbed Sheet Pan Chicken with Brussels Sprouts

PREP TIME: 15 MINUTES • COOK TIME: 30 MINUTES

Using bone-in chicken thighs with the skin makes them tender and drip with flavor. The herb seasoning mix can be prepared in advance and stored in an airtight container for up to 6 months. **SERVES 4**

1 teaspoon dried thyme

1 teaspoon dried basil

1 teaspoon freshly ground
   black pepper

½ teaspoon onion powder

½ teaspoon sea salt

½ teaspoon cayenne pepper

½ teaspoon paprika

Nonstick cooking spray, for
   coating the sheet pan

4 (8-ounce) bone-in, skin-on
   chicken thighs

2 pounds Brussels sprouts,
   trimmed and halved

⅓ cup extra-virgin olive oil

1. In a small bowl, stir together the thyme, basil, black pepper, onion powder, salt, cayenne, and paprika until blended.

2. Preheat the oven to 400°F. Line a large sheet pan with parchment paper, and coat with cooking spray.

3. In a large bowl, combine the chicken, Brussels sprouts, and oil.

4. Evenly sprinkle the herb seasoning mix over the chicken. Using clean hands, toss to coat.

5. Spread the chicken and Brussels sprouts evenly across the prepared sheet pan, leaving space between the ingredients.

6. Transfer the sheet pan to the oven, and bake for 30 minutes, or until the chicken reaches an internal temperature of 160°F. Remove from the oven. Let cool for 15 minutes.

STORAGE: Put in an airtight container. Refrigerate for up to 4 days, or freeze for up to 3 months.

THAWING AND REHEATING: Thaw in the refrigerator overnight. To reheat individual servings, put in a microwave-safe dish, and loosely cover with plastic wrap. Microwave on high power for 45 seconds. Stir and heat for 20 to 30 more seconds.

- -

Per Serving: Calories: 635; Total fat: 47g; Saturated fat: 10g; Protein: 35g; Total carbs: 22g; Fiber: 9g; Sugar: 5g; Sodium: 486mg

Cheesy Potato Soup

PREP TIME: 15 MINUTES • COOK TIME: 35 TO 40 MINUTES

This steamy soup, filled with chunks of potatoes and oozing with melted cheese, provides warmth and comfort on a chilly day. For a thicker soup, puree in a blender for 10 to 15 seconds. **SERVES 4**

2 tablespoons canola oil

1 cup chopped yellow onion

4 cups diced Russet potatoes

3 cups chicken broth

2 cups 2 percent milk

1 teaspoon sea salt

½ teaspoon paprika

½ teaspoon freshly ground black pepper

2 cups shredded sharp Cheddar cheese

4 bacon slices, cooked, drained, and crumbled (optional)

1. In a large saucepan, combine the oil and onion. Cook over medium heat, stirring often, for 5 to 7 minutes, or until the onion is tender and translucent.

2. Add the potatoes and broth. Bring to a boil.

3. Reduce the heat to low. Cover the pan, and simmer, stirring occasionally, for 20 minutes, or until the potatoes are tender.

4. Stir in the milk, salt, paprika, and pepper. Cook, stirring occasionally, for 5 minutes.

5. Add the cheese, and cook, stirring constantly, until the cheese is melted. Remove from the heat. Let cool for 15 to 20 minutes.

STORAGE: Put in an airtight container. Refrigerate for up to 4 days, or freeze for up to 3 months. Put 1 crumbled bacon slice in each of 4 (1-ounce) containers (if using), and refrigerate for up to 5 days, or freeze for up to 1 month.

THAWING AND REHEATING: Thaw in the refrigerator overnight. To reheat individual servings, put in a microwave-safe bowl, and cover with a paper towel. Microwave on 50 percent power for 1 minute. Stir and heat for 30 more seconds. Stir before serving.

SUBSTITUTION TIP: Beef broth or vegetable broth may be used instead of chicken broth.

Per Serving: Calories: 488; Total fat: 29g; Saturated fat: 13g; Protein: 21g; Total carbs: 38g; Fiber: 3g; Sugar: 9g; Sodium: 912mg

Skillet Spaghetti

PREP TIME: 20 MINUTES • COOK TIME: 30 MINUTES

Who knew a beefy spaghetti with homemade sauce could be so easy to prepare? This one-pot version requires minimal prep and, best of all, leaves only a few dishes to clean afterward. **SERVES 4**

2 tablespoons extra-virgin
  olive oil

1 cup chopped yellow onion

1 cup chopped green
  bell pepper

2 tablespoons minced garlic

1 pound 80/20 ground
  beef, cooked, crumbled,
  and drained

1 tablespoon Italian
  seasoning

1 teaspoon sea salt

4 cups beef broth

1 (14½-ounce) can diced
  tomatoes

1 (8-ounce) can tomato sauce

1 (12-ounce) package
  gluten-free spaghetti,
  broken into pieces

1. In a large saucepan, combine the oil, onion, bell pepper, and garlic. Cook over medium heat for 5 to 7 minutes, or until the onion is soft and translucent.

2. Add the beef, Italian seasoning, salt, broth, diced tomatoes with their juices, and tomato sauce. Stir to combine. Bring to a boil.

3. Reduce the heat to low. Add the spaghetti, stirring to make sure it is covered with sauce. Cook for 15 minutes, or until the spaghetti is al dente. Remove from the heat. Let cool for 15 minutes.

STORAGE: Put in an airtight container, making sure the pasta is covered with sauce. Refrigerate for up to 5 days, or freeze for up to 3 months.

THAWING AND REHEATING: Thaw in the refrigerator overnight. To reheat individual servings, put the spaghetti and sauce in a microwave-safe bowl, and add 1 tablespoon water. Microwave on 50 percent power for 1 minute. Stir and heat in 30-second intervals until warm, adding more water, if needed.

SUBSTITUTION TIP: Use crumbled cooked Italian sausage instead of ground beef. You can also puree 1 cup cooked carrots, and blend into the spaghetti while it simmers.

Per Serving: Calories: 725; Total fat: 32g; Saturated fat: 11g; Protein: 28g; Total carbs: 82g; Fiber: 7g; Sugar: 8g; Sodium: 784mg

Creole Black-Eyed Peas with Lentils

PREP TIME: 15 MINUTES • COOK TIME: 30 MINUTES

These black-eyed peas bring a taste of New Orleans to your kitchen. The "trinity" of Creole cooking—onion, bell pepper, and celery—along with a Creole seasoning blend are used to add flavor. SERVES 4

1 teaspoon ground cumin

1 teaspoon dried mustard

1 teaspoon sea salt

½ teaspoon curry powder

½ teaspoon chili powder

½ teaspoon freshly ground black pepper

3 tablespoons extra-virgin olive oil

1 cup chopped yellow onion

1 cup chopped green bell pepper

½ cup chopped celery

1 tablespoon minced garlic

1 (15½-ounce) can black-eyed peas, drained and rinsed

1 (14½-ounce) can diced tomatoes

3 cups cooked brown lentils

8 bacon slices, cooked, drained, and crumbled

1. To make the Creole spice mix, in a small bowl, stir together the cumin, dried mustard, salt, curry powder, chili powder, and pepper.

2. In a large saucepan, combine the oil, onion, bell pepper, celery, and garlic. Cook over medium-high heat for 5 to 7 minutes, or until the onion is soft and translucent.

3. Add the black-eyed peas, tomatoes with their juices, and Creole spice mix. Bring to a boil.

4. Reduce the heat to low. Simmer, stirring occasionally, for 20 minutes, or until the mixture has thickened. Remove from the heat.

5. Stir in the lentils and bacon. Let cool for 15 to 20 minutes.

STORAGE: Put in an airtight container. Refrigerate for up to 5 days, or freeze for up to 3 months.

THAWING AND REHEATING: Thaw in the refrigerator overnight. To reheat individual servings, put in a microwave-safe dish, and loosely cover with plastic wrap. Microwave on 50 percent power in 30-second intervals, stirring after each, until warm.

SUBSTITUTION TIP: Replace the black-eyed peas with drained canned black, kidney, navy, or pinto beans. Add 1 teaspoon red pepper flakes for more heat.

Per Serving: Calories: 485; Total fat: 19g; Saturated fat: 4g; Protein: 27g; Total carbs: 56g; Fiber: 21g; Sugar: 8g; Sodium: 997mg

Pumpkin Spice Muffins

PREP TIME: 20 MINUTES • COOK TIME: 15 TO 20 MINUTES

When fall arrives, so does pumpkin spice. It can be found every-where from coffee to these dense, flavorful muffins. They're delicious served as a breakfast or snack and taste even better with a pat of butter. MAKES 12 MUFFINS

Nonstick cooking spray, for coating the muffin tin

1¾ cups all-purpose gluten-free one-to-one baking flour

1½ cups sugar

1 teaspoon baking soda

1 teaspoon ground cinnamon

¾ teaspoon sea salt

½ teaspoon ground nutmeg

1 cup canned pumpkin

½ cup canola oil

2 large eggs, beaten

⅓ cup water

1. Preheat the oven to 400°F. Coat a 12-cup muffin tin with cooking spray.

2. In a large bowl, stir together the flour, sugar, baking soda, cinnamon, salt, and nutmeg until blended.

3. In a medium bowl, using a handheld mixer, blend the pumpkin, oil, eggs, and water on medium speed for 2 to 3 minutes.

4. To make the batter, pour the pumpkin mixture into the flour mixture. Mix until completely blended. Turn off the mixer.

5. Spoon ⅔ cup of the batter into each prepared muffin cup.

6. Transfer the muffin tin to the oven, and bake for 15 to 20 minutes, or until a knife inserted into the center of a muffin comes out clean. Remove from the oven. Let cool for 15 to 20 minutes.

STORAGE: Put the muffins in an airtight container. Store at room temperature for up to 3 days, refrigerate for up to 7 days, or freeze for up to 3 months.

THAWING AND REHEATING: Thaw in the refrigerator overnight. To reheat individual muffins, put on a microwave-safe plate, and cover with a paper towel. Microwave on high power for 30 seconds.

- -

Per Serving: Calories: 176; Total fat: 7g; Saturated fat: 1g; Protein: 2g; Total carbs: 27g; Fiber: 1g; Sugar: 17g; Sodium: 176mg

WINTER MENU:
Five-Recipe Meal Prep

It may be cold outside, but things are heating up in the kitchen, because these recipes are designed to be warm and filling. Egg salad gets an update with cheese and bacon, and pinto beans pair with pork chops in a Southwestern version of a traditional bean bake. Potatoes, quinoa, and winter squash mingle in a winter vegetable bake, and wild rice is the star of a thick, creamy soup. The menu rounds off with a breakfast burrito that's perfect for a handheld breakfast on the go. Pantry shoppers can substitute kidney beans or black beans for the pintos or buckwheat for the wild rice to speed up cooking time. Leftover jalapeños can be saved to use in the Cheese and Jalapeño Bake (page 56). Any extra bread can be made into bread crumbs and frozen for up to 3 months.

WINTER MENU:
Five-Recipe Meal Prep Shopping List

PRODUCE
Carrot (1)
Celery (1 bunch)
Onions, yellow (3)
Potatoes, Russet (2)
Sweet potatoes (2)

DAIRY AND EGGS
Butter, salted (8 ounces)
Cheese, Mexican-style, shredded
 (1 [8-ounce] bag)
Cheese, Cheddar, sharp, shredded
 (1 [8-ounce] bag)
Eggs, large (1 dozen)
Milk, whole (1 quart)
Sour cream, full-fat (1 [8-ounce] container)

MEAT
Bacon (1 [12-ounce] package)
Pork chops, bone-in (4 [8-ounce])
Sausage, pork, ground (1 pound)

FROZEN FOOD
Butternut squash, diced (1 [9-ounce]
 package)
Peas and carrots (1 [10-ounce] package)

CANNED AND BOTTLED
Beans, pinto (1 [15-ounce] can)
Broth, vegetable (1 [32-ounce] container)
Corn, whole kernel, Southwestern-style
 (1 [14½-ounce] can)
Jalapeños, pickled, sliced (1 [16-ounce] jar)
Mayonnaise, full-fat (1 [5½-ounce] container)
Tomatoes, diced, Southwestern-style
 (1 [14½-ounce] can)

PANTRY
Bread, gluten-free (1 loaf)
Quinoa (1 [1-pound] package)
Tortillas, flour, 8-inch, gluten-free
 (1 [8-count] package)
Wild rice (1 [1-pound] package)

CHECK YOUR PANTRY FOR . . .
All-purpose gluten-free one-to-one
baking flour, black peppercorns,
cayenne pepper, chili powder, dried
chives, dried oregano, garlic powder,
ground cumin, nonstick cooking
spray, onion powder, sea salt

Weekly Meal Chart

	BREAKFAST	LUNCH	DINNER
DAY 1	Sausage Breakfast Burrito	Egg Salad Sandwiches	Creamy Wild Rice Soup
DAY 2	Sausage Breakfast Burrito	Butternut Squash and Potato Bake	Egg Salad Sandwiches
DAY 3		Egg Salad Sandwiches	Creamy Wild Rice Soup
DAY 4	Sausage Breakfast Burrito	Pork Chop and Pinto Bean Bake	Egg Salad Sandwiches
DAY 5	Sausage Breakfast Burrito	Butternut Squash and Potato Bake	Creamy Wild Rice Soup
DAY 6		Pork Chop and Pinto Bean Bake	Butternut Squash and Potato Bake

STEP-BY-STEP PREP

1. Cook the wild rice. In a large saucepan, combine 2⅔ cups water and ⅔ cup wild rice. Bring to a boil over medium heat. Reduce the heat to low, cover the pan, and simmer for 45 minutes. Check to see if the rice is tender. If not, simmer for 5 to 10 more minutes. Remove from the heat. Drain any excess liquid.

2. Boil the eggs. In another large saucepan, combine 6 eggs and enough water to cover completely. Bring to a rolling boil over high heat. Turn off the heat. Cover the pan, and let the eggs sit for 12 minutes. Drain, and rinse the eggs with cool water. Peel and chop. Wash the pan.

3. Cook the quinoa. Rinse ⅔ cup quinoa in a strainer. In a large saucepan, combine 1 cup water and the quinoa. Bring to a boil over high heat. Reduce the heat

to low. Cover the pan, and simmer for 18 to 20 minutes, or until the quinoa is soft. Remove from the heat. Let rest for 5 minutes before using.

4. While the quinoa cooks, prep the vegetables for the week:

   ☐ *Drain 1 (16-ounce) jar jalapeños. Chop enough until you have ¼ cup chopped jalapeños, and set aside. Then dice enough jalapeños until you also have ½ cup diced.*

   ☐ *Chop 1 yellow onion, and set aside. Chop enough of the remaining onions until you have 2 (½-cup) portions; dice the remaining onion until you have ¾ cup.*

   ☐ *Dice enough celery to measure 1 (¾-cup) and 1 (1-cup) portion.*

   ☐ *Dice 2 sweet potatoes.*

   ☐ *Dice 2 Russet potatoes.*

   ☐ *Peel and dice 1 carrot.*

5. Cook the bacon. In a large skillet, cook 12 bacon slices (or just 7 if omitting from the Creamy Wild Rice Soup) over medium heat, turning every 2 to 3 minutes, for 7 to 10 minutes, or until they reach your desired crispness. Remove from the heat. Transfer to paper towels to drain and cool. Crumble the bacon. Wipe out the skillet.

6. Cook the sausage. In the same skillet, cook 1 pound ground pork sausage over medium heat, stirring to break up the meat, for 5 to 7 minutes, or until browned and no longer pink. Remove from the heat. Drain.

7. Make the bread crumbs. Set aside 8 gluten-free bread slices for the Egg Salad Sandwiches. Cut off the crusts from the remaining bread slices. Put the bread in a blender or food processor. Process for 5 to 10 seconds. Pour the crumbs into a small bowl.

8. Prepare the Butternut Squash and Potato Bake (page 88) as directed. Let cool for 15 minutes. Put in an airtight container. Refrigerate for up to 5 days, or freeze for up to 3 months.

9. Prepare the Pork Chop and Pinto Bean Bake (page 90) as directed. Let cool for 15 minutes. Put in an airtight container. Refrigerate for up to 3 days, or freeze for up to 3 months.

10. Prepare the Creamy Wild Rice Soup (page 91) as directed. Let

cool for 15 minutes. Put in an airtight container. Refrigerate for up to 5 days. This soup does not freeze well. Put 1 tablespoon crumbled bacon (if using) and 1 tablespoon shredded Cheddar cheese in each of 4 (2-ounce) containers. Refrigerate for up to 4 days, or freeze for up to 1 month.

11. Prepare the Sausage Breakfast Burrito (page 92) as directed. Let cool for 10 minutes. Wrap each burrito in parchment or wax paper before putting in an airtight container. Refrigerate for up to 4 days, or freeze for up to 2 months. Divide ¼ cup sour cream among 4 (1-ounce) containers, and refrigerate for up to 5 days.

12. Prepare the Egg Salad Sandwiches (page 93) as directed. Tightly wrap the sandwiches in aluminum foil, or put in resealable plastic bags. Refrigerate for up to 4 days. These sandwiches do not freeze well.

Butternut Squash and Potato Bake

PREP TIME: 20 MINUTES • COOK TIME: 40 TO 45 MINUTES

Most one-dish casseroles contain meat, but not this one! Sweet potatoes and winter squash are perked up with spices and cheese. Bread crumbs add crunch, while quinoa makes it a hearty meal. **SERVES 4**

Nonstick cooking spray, for coating the baking dish

1 teaspoon sea salt

1 teaspoon freshly ground black pepper

1 teaspoon dried oregano

1 teaspoon garlic powder

2 tablespoons salted butter

½ cup chopped yellow onion

1 (9-ounce) package frozen diced butternut squash

2 Russet potatoes, diced

2 sweet potatoes, diced

1 cup whole milk

1 tablespoon all-purpose gluten-free one-to-one baking flour

½ cup shredded sharp Cheddar cheese

2 cups cooked quinoa

Gluten-free bread crumbs, for topping

1. Preheat the oven to 350°F. Coat a 9-by-13-inch baking dish with cooking spray.

2. To make the spice mixture, in a small bowl, stir together the salt, pepper, oregano, and garlic powder.

3. In a medium skillet, combine the butter and onion. Cook over medium heat, stirring often, for 5 to 7 minutes, or until the onion is tender and translucent. Remove from the heat. Transfer to a large bowl.

4. Add the butternut squash, potatoes, and sweet potatoes to the bowl.

5. Stir in the spice mixture.

6. In a small bowl, whisk together the milk and flour until blended.

7. Add the cheese to the milk and flour.

8. Blend the cheese mixture into the squash mixture.

9. Stir in the quinoa.

10. Pour the mixture into the prepared baking dish.

11. Evenly sprinkle bread crumbs on top.

12. Transfer the baking dish to the oven, and bake for 30 to 35 minutes, or until the potatoes are tender when pierced with a fork. Remove from the oven. Let cool for 15 minutes.

STORAGE: Put in an airtight container. Refrigerate for up to 5 days, or freeze for up to 3 months.

THAWING AND REHEATING: Thaw in the refrigerator overnight. To reheat individual servings, put on a microwave-safe plate, and microwave on high power for 1 minute.

INGREDIENT TIP: Double the quinoa in the dish. Cook an additional 16-ounce package of quinoa according to the package directions. Let cool completely. Put in an airtight container, and freeze for up to 3 months to use in other dishes. Thaw in the refrigerator overnight.

Per Serving: Calories: 513; Total fat: 15g; Saturated fat: 8g; Protein: 16g; Total carbs: 83g; Fiber: 8g; Sugar: 10g; Sodium: 798mg

Pork and Pinto Bean Bake

PREP TIME: 20 MINUTES • COOK TIME: 35 MINUTES

Jalapeños add heat to this easy-to-prepare yet filling meat and bean dish. The Southwestern-style corn and tomatoes add even more chilies and spices to perk up a classic dish. **SERVES 4**

Nonstick cooking spray, for coating the baking dish

1 teaspoon garlic powder

1 teaspoon chili powder

1 teaspoon ground cumin

¼ teaspoon cayenne pepper

1 (15-ounce) can pinto beans, drained and rinsed

1 (15-ounce) can Southwestern-style whole kernel corn, drained

1 (14½-ounce) can Southwestern-style diced tomatoes

½ cup diced pickled jalapeño peppers

1 tablespoon all-purpose gluten-free one-to-one baking flour

½ cup whole milk

2 tablespoons salted butter

½ cup chopped yellow onion

4 (8-ounce) bone-in pork chops

1. Preheat the oven to 350°F. Coat a 9-by-13-inch baking dish with cooking spray.

2. In a large bowl, stir together the garlic powder, chili powder, cumin, and cayenne.

3. Stir in the beans, corn, tomatoes with their juices, and jalapeños until blended.

4. To make a slurry, in a small bowl, whisk together the flour and milk until blended. Stir the slurry into the bean mixture.

5. In an oven-safe skillet, combine the butter and onion. Cook over medium heat, stirring often, for 5 to 7 minutes, or until the onion is tender and translucent.

6. Add the bean mixture.

7. Place the pork chops on top of the bean mixture.

8. Transfer the skillet to the oven, and bake for 30 to 35 minutes, or until the chops are browned and reach an internal temperature of 145°F. Remove from the oven. Let cool for 15 minutes.

STORAGE: Put in an airtight container. Refrigerate for up to 3 days, or freeze for up to 3 months.

THAWING AND REHEATING: Thaw in the refrigerator overnight. To reheat individual servings, put on a microwave-safe dish. Microwave on high power for 30 seconds. Flip the pork chops, and stir the beans. Heat for 15 to 30 more seconds.

Per Serving: Calories: 486; Total fat: 22g; Saturated fat: 9g; Protein: 38g; Total carbs: 36g; Fiber: 5g; Sugar: 7g; Sodium: 461mg

Creamy Wild Rice Soup

PREP TIME: 1 HOUR • COOK TIME: 20 MINUTES

Wild rice takes time to cook, but it's worth it for a bowl of this thick, rich soup. Flavored with chives and topped with bacon and cheese, this is perfect for any time you need a warm pick-me-up. **SERVES 4**

2 tablespoons salted butter

1 yellow onion, chopped

1 carrot, diced

1 cup diced celery

¼ cup all-purpose gluten-free one-to-one baking flour

¼ teaspoon sea salt

¼ teaspoon freshly ground black pepper

1 teaspoon dried chives

1 teaspoon garlic powder

1 (10-ounce) package frozen peas and carrots

4 cups vegetable broth

2 cups cooked wild rice

½ cup whole milk

5 bacon slices, cooked, drained, and crumbled (optional)

¼ cup shredded sharp Cheddar cheese (optional)

1. In a large saucepan, combine the butter, onion, carrot, and celery. Cook over medium heat, stirring often, for 5 to 7 minutes, or until the onion is tender and translucent.

2. Stir in the flour until blended.

3. Add the salt, pepper, chives, garlic powder, peas and carrots, broth, and wild rice. Bring to a boil. Cook, stirring constantly, for 2 minutes.

4. Reduce the heat to low. Stir in the milk. Cook, stirring often, for 3 to 5 minutes, or until slightly thickened. Remove from the heat. Let cool for 15 minutes.

STORAGE: Put in an airtight container. Refrigerate for up to 5 days. This soup does not freeze well. Put 1 tablespoon crumbled bacon (if using) and 1 tablespoon shredded Cheddar cheese (if using) in each of 4 (2-ounce) containers. Refrigerate for up to 4 days, or freeze for up to 1 month.

THAWING AND REHEATING: Thaw in the refrigerator overnight. To reheat individual servings, put the soup in a microwave-safe bowl, and cover. Microwave on high power for 30 to 45 seconds. Stir and heat for 15 to 20 more seconds, if needed.

Per Serving: Calories: 242; Total fat: 8g; Saturated fat: 4g; Protein: 8g; Total carbs: 38g; Fiber: 6g; Sugar: 4g; Sodium: 295mg

Sausage Breakfast Burrito

PREP TIME: 20 MINUTES • COOK TIME: 5 MINUTES

These burritos can go from mild to wild. Adjust the heat by using hot or mild sausage, along with mild, medium, or hot green chilies. SERVES 4

½ teaspoon sea salt

½ teaspoon garlic powder

½ teaspoon onion powder

½ teaspoon freshly ground black pepper

6 large eggs, beaten

½ cup whole milk

¼ cup chopped pickled jalapeño peppers

1 cup shredded Mexican-style cheese

2 tablespoons salted butter

1 pound ground pork sausage, cooked, drained, and crumbled

8 (8-inch) gluten-free flour tortillas

¼ cup full-fat sour cream

1. In a small bowl, stir together the salt, garlic powder, onion powder, and pepper.

2. Stir in the eggs, milk, jalapeños, and cheese until well blended.

3. In a medium skillet, combine the butter and egg mixture. Cook over medium-high heat, stirring constantly, for 3 to 5 minutes, or until the eggs are light and fluffy.

4. Stir in the sausage. Remove from the heat.

5. Put the tortillas on a work surface.

6. Spoon ½ cup of the egg-sausage mixture into each tortilla.

7. Roll the tortillas burrito-style. Let cool for 10 minutes.

8. Serve the burritos with the sour cream.

STORAGE: Wrap each burrito in parchment or wax paper before putting in an airtight container. Refrigerate for up to 4 days, or freeze for up to 2 months. Put 1 tablespoon sour cream in each of 4 (1-ounce) containers, and refrigerate for up to 5 days.

THAWING AND REHEATING: Thaw in the refrigerator overnight. To reheat individual burritos, put on a microwave-safe plate, and cover with a damp paper towel. Microwave on 50 percent power for 45 seconds to 1 minute. Heat for 15 to 30 more seconds, if needed.

SUBSTITUTION TIP: Replace the sausage with 1 (12-ounce) package bacon, cooked, drained, and crumbled, or 1 pound crumbled cooked Italian sausage.

Per Serving: Calories: 967; Total fat: 64g; Saturated fat: 28g; Protein: 45g; Total carbs: 60g; Fiber: 10g; Sugar: 10g; Sodium: 2,440mg

Egg Salad Sandwiches

PREP TIME: 20 MINUTES

Take ho-hum egg salad from blah and boring to tempting and tasty with the addition of bacon and cheese. Serve this without the bread for a light lunch or snack. **SERVES 4**

⅔ cup full-fat mayonnaise

½ teaspoon sea salt

½ teaspoon freshly ground black pepper

¾ cup diced yellow onion

¾ cup diced celery

6 hard-boiled eggs, peeled and chopped

¼ cup shredded sharp Cheddar cheese

7 bacon slices, cooked, drained, and crumbled

8 gluten-free bread slices

1. In a large bowl, stir together the mayonnaise, salt, pepper, onion, celery, and eggs.

2. Stir in the cheese and bacon.

3. Put 4 bread slices on a work surface.

4. Gently spread ¾ cup of the egg salad onto each slice.

5. Top the egg salad with another slice of bread.

STORAGE: Tightly wrap the sandwiches in aluminum foil, or put in resealable plastic bags. Refrigerate for up to 4 days. Do not freeze.

INGREDIENT TIP: Although the whites of hard-boiled eggs become tough and rubbery when frozen, the yolks do not. Hard-boiled egg yolks can be frozen for up to 3 months. Egg yolks can be used to make deviled eggs, added to salads, or grated over pasta.

- -

Per Serving: Calories: 629; Total fat: 49g; Saturated fat: 11g; Protein: 20g; Total carbs: 26g; Fiber: 6g; Sugar: 3g; Sodium: 1,180mg

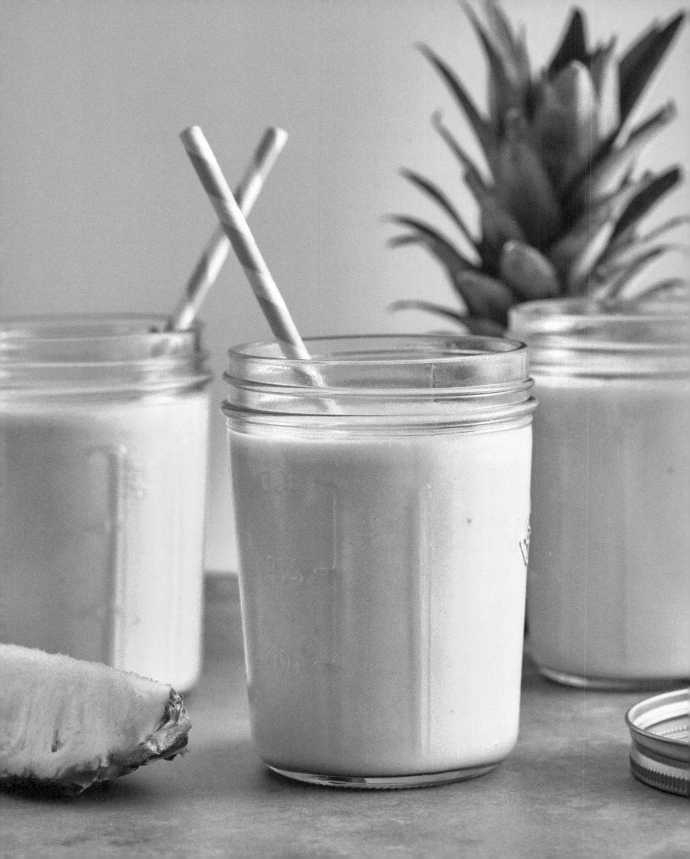

Stepping Up to Six: Six-Recipe Meal Preps

We've stepped up to six recipes, which should require about 3 hours in the kitchen. Our new addition will be either a snack or dessert. If any of the dessert or snack recipes are not your thing, feel free to replace them with another recipe from chapter 8. This week features a variety of comforting foods—from a savory omelet to home-style chicken and potatoes in tomato sauce. The cool layered salad offers an unusual but tempting combination of broccoli, bacon, fruit, and seeds. We've even taken a Creole favorite—shrimp etouffée—and made it easier to prepare with a simplified roux. Want to plan ahead? Peel, slice, and freeze the bananas used for the "nice" cream. Shop your pantry before going to the store. Substitute quinoa or buckwheat for the rice and walnuts for the pecans.

‹‹ Peach and Pineapple Smoothie, page 118

SPRING MENU:
Six-Recipe Prep Shopping List

PRODUCE
Bananas (5)
Bell pepper, green (1)
Broccoli (1 large head)
Carrots (2)
Celery (1 bunch)
Chives (1 bunch)
Garlic (1 head)
Lemon (1)
Mushrooms, cremini (1 [8-ounce] container)
Onion, red (1)
Onions, yellow (4)
Parsley (1 bunch)
Potatoes, Russet (5)

DAIRY AND EGGS
Butter, salted (8 ounces)
Cheese, Cheddar, mild, shredded
  (1 [8-ounce] bag)
Eggs, large (1 dozen)
Milk, whole (1 pint)

MEAT
Bacon (1 [12-ounce] package)
Chicken, breasts, boneless, skinless (2 pounds)

FROZEN FOOD
Shrimp, medium, peeled, deveined, tails off
  (1 pound)
Squash, yellow (1 [10-ounce] package)

CANNED AND BOTTLED
Broth, chicken (1 [14½-ounce] can)
Broth, vegetable (1 [32-ounce] container)
Mayonnaise, full-fat (1 [5½-ounce] container)
Olives, green, sliced (1 [4-ounce] jar)
Tomatoes, Italian-style, diced
  (1 [28-ounce] can)

PANTRY
Cocoa powder, unsweetened (1 [8-ounce]
  container)
Coffee powder, instant mocha
  (1 [6½-ounce] box)
Pecans (1 cup)
Raisins (1 cup)
Rice, long-grain, white (1 [1-pound] package)
Sunflower seeds (1 cup)

CHECK YOUR PANTRY FOR . . .
All-purpose gluten-free one-to-one baking flour, bay leaf, black peppercorns, canola oil, cayenne pepper, cornstarch, distilled white vinegar, dried basil, dried marjoram, dried thyme, extra-virgin olive oil, gluten-free hot pepper sauce, nonstick cooking spray, prepared mustard, sea salt, seasoned salt, sugar, vanilla extract

Weekly Meal Chart

	BREAKFAST	LUNCH	DINNER	DESSERT
DAY 1	Herb, Cheese, and Mushroom Omelet	Squash and Potato Bisque	Layered Broccoli Salad	Chocolate, Pecan, and Mocha "Nice" Cream
DAY 2	Herb, Cheese, and Mushroom Omelet	Layered Broccoli Salad	Shrimp Etouffée	Chocolate, Pecan, and Mocha "Nice" Cream
DAY 3	Herb, Cheese, and Mushroom Omelet	Smothered Chicken and Potatoes	Layered Broccoli Salad	Chocolate, Pecan, and Mocha "Nice" Cream
DAY 4		Layered Broccoli Salad	Squash and Potato Bisque	Chocolate, Pecan, and Mocha "Nice" Cream
DAY 5	Herb, Cheese, and Mushroom Omelet	Shrimp Etouffée	Smothered Chicken and Potatoes	Chocolate, Pecan, and Mocha "Nice" Cream
DAY 6		Smothered Chicken and Potatoes	Shrimp Etouffée	

STEP-BY-STEP PREP

1. Peel and slice 5 bananas. Put in an airtight container, and freeze.

2. Prep the vegetables for the week:

   ☐ *Chop 4 yellow onions, and divide into 4 (1-cup) portions.*

   ☐ *Thinly slice 1 red onion.*

   ☐ *Chop 1 head broccoli.*

   ☐ *Seed and chop enough green bell pepper to measure ½ cup.*

   ☐ *Dice 5 Russet potatoes.*

   ☐ *Peel and thinly slice 2 carrots.*

- ☐ *Slice 8 ounces mushrooms.*
- ☐ *Chop enough celery to measure 1 cup.*
- ☐ *Mince enough garlic to measure 3 tablespoons.*
- ☐ *Mince 1 bunch parsley.*
- ☐ *Mince 1 bunch chives.*
- ☐ *Juice enough lemon to measure 1 tablespoon juice.*

3. Cook the rice. In a large saucepan, combine 2 cups water and 1 cup long-grain white rice. Bring to a boil over high heat. Reduce the heat to low, cover the pan, and simmer for 15 minutes, or until tender. Remove from the heat. Let rest for 10 minutes.

4. Cook the bacon. In a large skillet, cook 12 bacon slices (or just 8 if omitting from the Squash and Potato Bisque) over medium heat, turning every 2 to 3 minutes, for 7 to 10 minutes, or until they reach your desired crispness. Remove from the heat. Transfer to paper towels to drain and cool. Crumble the bacon.

5. Prepare the Squash and Potato Bisque (page 100) as directed. Let cool for 20 minutes. Put in an airtight container. Refrigerate for up to 5 days, or freeze for up to 3 months. Chives and crumbled, cooked bacon can be used for topping. Put 1½ teaspoons minced chives and 1 crumbled bacon slice (if using) in each of 4 (1-ounce) containers, and refrigerate for up to 5 days.

6. Prepare the Shrimp Etouffée (page 101) as directed. Let cool for 20 minutes. Store in an airtight container. Refrigerate for up to 4 days, or freeze for up to 1 month. Put 1 tablespoon of the parsley-chive mixture in each of 4 (1-ounce) containers. Refrigerate for up to 2 weeks.

7. Prepare the Smothered Chicken and Potatoes (page 103) as directed. Let cool for 20 minutes. Put in an airtight container. Refrigerate for up to 4 days, or freeze for up to 3 months. Put 1 tablespoon of the parsley-chive mixture in each of 4 (1-ounce) containers. Refrigerate for up to 2 weeks. Divide ¼ cup Cheddar cheese among 4 (1-ounce) containers (if using). Refrigerate for up to 1 week, or freeze for up to 3 months.

8. Prepare the Herb, Cheese, and Mushroom Omelet (page 105) as directed. Let cool for 15 minutes. Tightly wrap each omelet in wax paper or parchment paper before

putting in an airtight container. Refrigerate for up to 5 days, or freeze for up to 2 months.

9. Prepare the Layered Broccoli Salad (page 107) as directed. Seal the lids. Divide the dressing among 4 (1-ounce) containers. Refrigerate the salads and dressing for up to 5 days. Do not freeze.

10. Remove the bananas from the freezer. Prepare the Chocolate, Pecan, and Mocha "Nice" Cream (page 108) as directed. Put in an airtight container, and freeze for up to 2 months. Let sit at room temperature for 5 to 10 minutes before eating.

Squash and Potato Bisque

PREP TIME: 15 MINUTES • COOK TIME: 45 MINUTES

Frozen yellow squash and Russet potatoes blend to create this creamy smooth soup with true down-home flavor. Top with leftover crumbled cooked bacon or chopped fresh chives. **SERVES 4**

7 tablespoons salted butter

1 cup chopped yellow onion

2 Russet potatoes, diced

2 carrots, thinly sliced

1 (10-ounce) package frozen yellow squash

4 cups vegetable broth

¼ teaspoon sea salt

1 teaspoon gluten-free hot pepper sauce

1 tablespoon dried thyme

1 cup whole milk

2 tablespoons minced fresh chives

4 bacon slices, cooked, drained, and crumbled

1. In a large saucepan, combine the butter, onion, potatoes, and carrots. Cook over medium-high heat, stirring often, for 5 to 7 minutes, or until the onion is translucent.

2. Reduce the heat to medium-low. Add the squash, broth, salt, hot sauce, and thyme. Stir to combine. Cover the pan, and simmer, stirring occasionally, for 25 to 30 minutes, or until the vegetables are fork-tender.

3. Carefully pour half of the soup into a food processor or blender. Process for 5 to 10 seconds, or until pureed. Pour into a large bowl. Repeat with the remaining soup.

4. Return the pureed soup to the saucepan. Alternatively, use an immersion blender to blend the soup in the pan.

5. Add the milk. Bring to a boil over high heat, stirring constantly. Boil for 1 minute. Remove from the heat. Let cool for 20 minutes. Serve with the chives and bacon.

STORAGE: Put soup in an airtight container. Refrigerate for up to 5 days, or freeze for up to 3 months.

THAWING AND REHEATING: Thaw in the refrigerator overnight. To reheat individual servings, put the soup in a microwave-safe dish, and cover with a paper towel. Microwave on 50 percent power for 30 seconds. Stir and heat for 30 to 45 more seconds. Stir before serving.

- -

Per Serving: Calories: 405; Total fat: 22g; Saturated fat: 14g; Protein: 7g; Total carbs: 47g; Fiber: 5g; Sugar: 7g; Sodium: 398mg

Shrimp Etouffée

PREP TIME: 25 MINUTES • COOK TIME: 35 MINUTES

This classic Creole dish can be found on almost every corner in New Orleans. Our simple roux replaces the usual slow-cooked roux. Adjust the hot sauce to your desired heat level. SERVES 4

1 tablespoon all-purpose gluten-free one-to-one baking flour

1 tablespoon salted butter, melted

1 tablespoon prepared mustard

1 tablespoon gluten-free hot pepper sauce

1 teaspoon cayenne pepper

½ teaspoon sea salt

3 tablespoons minced fresh parsley, divided

1 (14½-ounce) can Italian-style diced tomatoes

½ cup canola oil

1 cup chopped celery

1 cup chopped yellow onion

½ cup chopped green bell pepper

2 tablespoons minced garlic

1 bay leaf

1 pound frozen medium shrimp, peeled, deveined, tails removed

1 tablespoon freshly squeezed lemon juice

3 cups cooked long-grain white rice

2 tablespoons minced fresh chives

1. In a small bowl, whisk together the flour and butter until blended.

2. In another small bowl, stir together the mustard, hot sauce, cayenne, salt, 1 tablespoon of parsley, and the tomatoes with their juices.

3. In a large skillet, combine the oil, celery, onion, bell pepper, and garlic. Cook over medium heat, stirring occasionally, for 5 to 7 minutes, or until the vegetables are tender and the onion is translucent.

4. Add the tomato and spice mixture and bay leaf.

5. Sprinkle the flour mixture into the skillet, and cook, stirring constantly, for 3 minutes, or until the sauce has slightly thickened.

6. Reduce the heat to low. Simmer, stirring occasionally, for 20 minutes, or until the sauce has reduced by one-fourth.

7. Add the shrimp, and cook for 5 minutes, or until cooked through.

8. Remove and discard the bay leaf.

9. Stir in the lemon juice and rice. Remove from the heat. Let cool for 20 minutes.

10. In a small bowl, stir together the remaining 2 tablespoons of parsley and the chives.

11. Serve the shrimp and rice with the parsley and chives.

CONTINUED ⟶

STORAGE: Put in an airtight container. Refrigerate for up to 4 days, or freeze for up to 1 month. Put 1 tablespoon of the parsley-chive mixture in each of 4 (1-ounce) containers. Refrigerate for up to 2 weeks.

THAWING AND REHEATING: Thaw in the refrigerator overnight. To reheat individual servings, put in a microwave-safe container, and loosely cover with a paper towel. Microwave on 50 percent power for 1 minute. Stir and heat for 30 more seconds, if needed. Stir before serving.

SUBSTITUTION TIP: One pound of crawfish meat can be substituted for the shrimp.

Per Serving: Calories: 561; Total fat: 32g; Saturated fat: 4g; Protein: 21g; Total carbs: 47g; Fiber: 4g; Sugar: 5g; Sodium: 1,030mg

Smothered Chicken and Potatoes

PREP TIME: 20 MINUTES • COOK TIME: 25 MINUTES

A rich herb-seasoned tomato sauce makes this baked chicken and potato dish a true comfort. Replace the water with leftover chicken broth, if desired. Any leftover cheese can be sprinkled over the chicken before serving. SERVES 4

Nonstick cooking spray, for coating the baking dish

1 (14½-ounce) can Italian-style diced tomatoes

4 tablespoons minced fresh parsley, divided

1 tablespoon minced garlic

½ teaspoon seasoned salt

½ teaspoon dried basil

½ teaspoon dried marjoram

½ cup chicken broth

1 teaspoon cornstarch

2 teaspoons water

2 pounds boneless, skinless chicken breasts

1 cup chopped yellow onion

3 Russet potatoes, diced

2 tablespoons minced fresh chives

¼ cup shredded mild Cheddar cheese (optional)

1. Preheat the oven to 350°F. Coat a 9-by-13-inch baking dish with cooking spray.

2. To make the tomato sauce, in a medium bowl, stir together the tomatoes with their juices, 2 tablespoons of parsley, the garlic, seasoned salt, basil, marjoram, and broth until blended.

3. To make a slurry, in a small cup, whisk together the cornstarch and water until blended.

4. Stir the slurry into the tomato sauce.

5. Put the chicken, onion, and potatoes in the prepared baking dish.

6. Cover with the tomato sauce.

7. Transfer the baking dish to the oven, and bake for 25 minutes, or until the chicken reaches an internal temperature of 165°F and the potatoes pierce easily with a fork. Remove from the oven. Let cool for 20 minutes.

8. In a small bowl, stir together the remaining 2 tablespoons of parsley and the chives.

9. Serve the chicken and potatoes with the parsley, chives, and cheese (if using).

STORAGE: Put in an airtight container. Refrigerate for up to 4 days, or freeze for up to 3 months. Put 1 tablespoon of the parsley-chive mixture in each of 4 (1-ounce) containers. Refrigerate for up to 2 weeks. Divide the

CONTINUED ⟶

Cheddar cheese among 4 (1-ounce) containers (if using). Refrigerate for up to 1 week, or freeze for up to 3 months.

THAWING AND REHEATING: Thaw in the refrigerator overnight. To reheat individual servings, put in a microwave-safe container, and loosely cover with a paper towel. Microwave on 50 percent power for 1 minute. Stir and heat for 30 more seconds, if needed.

SUBSTITUTION TIP: Chicken thighs can also be used. Increase the baking time to 30 to 35 minutes.

Per Serving: Calories: 507; Total fat: 4g; Saturated fat: 1g; Protein: 58g; Total carbs: 59g; Fiber: 7g; Sugar: 6g; Sodium: 435mg

Herb, Cheese, and Mushroom Omelet

PREP TIME: 20 MINUTES • COOK TIME: 50 MINUTES

This omelet, made with fresh herbs, fresh mushrooms, and Cheddar cheese, is a savory start to the day. Leftover bell pepper can be added to the onion and mushroom mixture while sautéing. **SERVES 4**

2 tablespoons extra-virgin olive oil

1 (8-ounce) container cremini mushrooms, sliced

1 cup chopped yellow onion

12 large eggs

¼ cup whole milk

1 teaspoon sea salt

½ teaspoon freshly ground black pepper

3 tablespoons minced fresh parsley

3 tablespoons minced fresh chives

½ cup shredded mild Cheddar cheese

8 tablespoons (1 stick) salted butter, divided

1. In a medium skillet, combine the oil, mushrooms, and onion. Cook over medium heat, stirring often, for 5 to 7 minutes, or until the onion is tender and translucent. Remove from the heat.

2. In a large bowl, whisk together the eggs, milk, salt, and pepper until blended.

3. Add the parsley, chives, mushroom-onion mixture, and cheese to the bowl. Whisk to combine.

4. Wipe out the skillet used to cook the mushrooms. In the skillet, melt 2 tablespoons of the butter over medium heat.

5. Add one-fourth of the egg mixture. Cook, lifting the edges using a spatula to allow uncooked egg to flow underneath, for 7 to 10 minutes, or until creamy and set.

6. Using the spatula, fold the omelet in half. Slide the spatula underneath the omelet, and flip onto a plate. Repeat with the remaining butter and egg mixture. This should make 4 omelets. Turn off the heat. Let cool for 15 minutes.

STORAGE: Tightly wrap each omelet in wax paper or parchment paper before placing in an airtight container. Refrigerate for up to 5 days, or freeze for up to 2 months.

CONTINUED ⟶

THAWING AND REHEATING: Thaw in the refrigerator overnight. To reheat individual servings, put the omelet on a microwave-safe dish, and loosely cover with a paper towel. Microwave on high power for 1 minute. Flip the omelet, and heat for 30 more seconds, if needed.

SUBSTITUTION TIP: Use 1 tablespoon dried chives and 1 tablespoon dried parsley instead of the fresh herbs.

Per Serving: Calories: 575; Total fat: 50g; Saturated fat: 23g; Protein: 25g; Total carbs: 8g; Fiber: 1g; Sugar: 4g; Sodium: 981mg

Layered Broccoli Salad

PREP TIME: 20 MINUTES

Crunchy broccoli and crisp bacon give this salad a pleasing crunch, while the raisins and green olives add sweet and sour notes. Have leftover pecans? Add them to the salad. **SERVES 4**

For the salad

1 large head
   broccoli, chopped

1 red onion, thinly sliced

1 cup raisins

1 cup sunflower seeds

1 (4-ounce) jar sliced green
   olives, drained

8 bacon slices, cooked,
   drained, and crumbled

½ cup shredded mild
   Cheddar cheese

For the dressing

½ cup full-fat mayonnaise

2 tablespoons distilled
   white vinegar

¼ cup sugar

To make the salad

1. In each of 4 (1-pint) Mason jars, layer ½ cup of broccoli, ¼ cup of onion, ¼ cup of raisins, ¼ cup of sunflower seeds, and 1 tablespoon of olives.

2. Divide the bacon and cheese among the jars. To prepare 1 large salad, in a large bowl or on a serving platter, layer the ingredients as listed.

To make the dressing

3. In a small bowl, whisk together the mayonnaise, vinegar, and sugar until blended.

STORAGE: Divide the dressing among 4 (1-ounce) containers. Refrigerate the salads and dressing for up to 5 days. Do not freeze.

SUBSTITUTION TIP: Replace the broccoli with chopped cauliflower. Create your own salad with any of the following toppings: 1 cup chopped almonds, 1 cup Cajun-Spiced Pumpkin Seeds (page 188), or ½ cup crumbled blue cheese. Italian Dressing (page 182) can replace the mayonnaise-based dressing here.

Per Serving: Calories: 773; Total fat: 55g; Saturated fat: 10g; Protein: 21g; Total carbs: 57g; Fiber: 8g; Sugar: 38g; Sodium: 995mg

Chocolate, Pecan, and Mocha "Nice" Cream

PREP TIME: 10 MINUTES

Bananas replace the cream and sugar used in traditional ice cream recipes in this creamy frozen treat. Add more or less cocoa powder and instant coffee powder to suit your taste. **SERVES 5**

5 bananas, peeled, sliced, and frozen

2 teaspoons vanilla extract

¼ cup unsweetened cocoa powder

¼ cup instant mocha coffee powder

1 cup pecans

½ teaspoon sea salt

⅓ cup whole milk

1. In a high-speed blender or food processor, combine the bananas, vanilla, cocoa powder, coffee powder, pecans, salt, and milk. Pulse for 20 seconds.

2. Using a spatula, scrape down any chunks of banana, and pulse for 10 to 15 seconds, or until blended.

STORAGE: Put in an airtight container. Freeze for up to 2 months.

THAWING AND REHEATING: Let sit at room temperature for 5 to 10 minutes before eating.

VARIATION TIP:

BERRY-CHOCOLATE "NICE" CREAM: Replace the mocha coffee powder and pecans with 1 cup frozen mixed berries.

CHOCOLATE-COCONUT "NICE" CREAM: Replace the mocha coffee powder with ¾ cup flaked coconut.

FRENCH VANILLA AND ALMOND "NICE" CREAM: Replace the cocoa powder and mocha coffee powder with ½ cup French vanilla instant coffee powder. Substitute 1 cup almonds for the pecans.

Per Serving: Calories: 290; Total fat: 17g; Saturated fat: 2g; Protein: 5g; Total carbs: 37g; Fiber: 6g; Sugar: 19g; Sodium: 258mg

SUMMER MENU:
Six-Recipe Meal Prep

This summer prep delivers a healthy snack, a fruity salad, a refreshing smoothie, and another taste of New Orleans with a Creole "Crabmeat" Pie (page 113). And, who says you can't eat pie for breakfast? The quiche-like texture makes this pie good at any meal. Trail mix is shelf stable for up to 2 weeks and can be packed in individual air-tight containers for a quick on-the-go snack. Double this easy recipe to keep a supply of trail mix steady. Shop your pantry, and replace quinoa with lentils, millet, or a rice of your choice. Check your refrigerator, and replace the Cheddar cheese with your favorite cheese. Leftover ingredients can be used to create new recipes or added to others during prep. For example, leftover bacon can be used in Twice-Baked Potatoes (page 115).

SUMMER MENU:
Six-Recipe Meal Prep Shopping List

PRODUCE
Bananas (3)
Bell peppers, green (2)
Celery (1 bunch)
Mixed greens (1 [1-pound] package)
Onions, yellow (3)
Oranges, for juice (2)
Potatoes, Russet, large (4)
Strawberries (1 [1-pound] package)

DAIRY AND EGGS
Butter, salted (8 ounces)
Cheese, Cheddar, sharp, shredded
    (1 [8-ounce] bag)
Cheese, goat, crumbled (1 [3-ounce]
    package)
Eggs, large (1 half dozen)
Milk, whole (1 pint)
Yogurt, full-fat, plain (1 [8-ounce] container)
Yogurt, full-fat, vanilla (1 [1-pound]
    container)

MEAT
Bacon (1 [12-ounce] package)
Beef, steak, sirloin, boneless (1 pound)
Crab, gluten-free, imitation (1 [8-ounce]
    package)

FROZEN FOOD
Piecrust, gluten-free, deep dish, 9-inch (1)

CANNED AND BOTTLED
Mandarin orange slices (1 [11-ounce] can)
Peach slices in juice (1 [15-ounce] can)
Pineapple chunks in juice (1 [15-ounce] can)
Tomatoes, diced (1 [14½-ounce] can)

PANTRY
Dried fruit, mixed (1 [1-pound] package)
Nuts, mixed (1 [10½-ounce] container)
Pumpkin seeds (1 [8-ounce] package)
Quinoa (1 [16-ounce] package)
Sunflower seeds (1 [8-ounce] package)

CHECK YOUR PANTRY FOR . . .
Black peppercorns, cayenne pepper,
cornstarch, distilled white vinegar,
dried chives, extra-virgin olive oil,
garlic powder, gluten-free soy sauce
or tamari, ground ginger, nonstick
cooking spray, paprika, sea salt, sugar

Weekly Meal Chart

	BREAKFAST	LUNCH	DINNER	SNACK
DAY 1	Peach and Pineapple Smoothie	Fruity Mixed Greens Salad	Creole "Crabmeat" Pie	Fruit, Seed, and Nut Trail Mix
DAY 2	Peach and Pineapple Smoothie	Pepper Steak	Fruity Mixed Greens Salad	Fruit, Seed, and Nut Trail Mix
DAY 3	Creole "Crabmeat" Pie	Twice-Baked Potatoes	Pepper Steak	Fruit, Seed, and Nut Trail Mix
DAY 4	Peach and Pineapple Smoothie	Creole "Crabmeat" Pie	Fruity Mixed Greens Salad	Fruit, Seed, and Nut Trail Mix
DAY 5	Peach and Pineapple Smoothie	Fruity Mixed Greens Salad	Twice-Baked Potatoes	Fruit, Seed, and Nut Trail Mix
DAY 6		Pepper Steak	Creole "Crabmeat" Pie	Fruit, Seed, and Nut Trail Mix

STEP-BY-STEP PREP

1. Peel and slice 3 bananas. Put in an airtight container, and freeze.

2. Rinse 1 cup quinoa in a strainer. In a large saucepan, combine 1¾ cups water and the quinoa. Bring to a boil over high heat. Reduce the heat to low, cover the pan, and simmer for 18 to 20 minutes.

Remove from the heat. Let rest for 5 minutes before using.

3. While the quinoa cooks, prep the vegetables for the week:

   ☐ *Chop 2 yellow onions, and divide into 2 equal portions. Chop enough of the third onion to measure ½ cup.*

☐ *Chop enough celery to measure ½ cup.*

☐ *Seed and chop 1 green bell pepper. Set aside. Seed and chop enough of the second bell pepper to measure 1 cup.*

☐ *Hull and slice 1 pound strawberries.*

☐ *Juice enough oranges to measure ½ cup juice.*

☐ *Wash and dry 1 pound Russet potatoes.*

4. Cook the bacon. In a large skillet, cook 12 bacon slices (or just 10, if omitting from the Twice-Baked Potatoes) over medium heat, turning every 2 to 3 minutes, for 7 to 10 minutes, or until they reach your desired crispness. Remove from the heat. Transfer to paper towels to drain and cool. Crumble the bacon.

5. Preheat the oven to 325°F.

6. Blind-bake the piecrust. Using a fork, prick holes across the bottom and sides of the piecrust. Put in the oven, and bake for 10 minutes, or until the crust has lightly browned. Remove from the oven, leaving the oven on.

7. Prepare the Creole "Crabmeat" Pie (page 113) as directed. Let cool for 20 minutes. Tightly wrap the pie in aluminum foil, or put in an

airtight container. Refrigerate for up to 5 days, or freeze for up to 2 months.

8. Prepare the Pepper Steak (page 114) as directed. Let cool for 20 minutes. Put in an airtight container. Refrigerate for up to 4 days, or freeze for up to 3 months.

9. Increase the oven temperature to 350°F. Prepare the Twice-Baked Potatoes (page 115) as directed. Let cool for 20 minutes. Tightly wrap each potato in foil, or put in airtight containers. Refrigerate for up to 5 days, or freeze for up to 3 months.

10. Prepare the Fruity Mixed Greens Salad (page 117) as directed. Refrigerate for up to 5 days. Divide the dressing among 4 (1-ounce) containers, and refrigerate for up to 5 days. The salad should not be frozen.

11. Prepare the Peach and Pineapple Smoothie (page 118) as directed. Seal the jars, and refrigerate for up to 4 days, or freeze for up to 2 months.

12. Prepare the Fruit, Seed, and Nut Trail Mix (page 119) as directed. Put in an airtight container. Store at room temperature for up to 2 weeks, or freeze for up to 3 months.

Creole "Crabmeat" Pie

PREP TIME: 20 MINUTES • COOK TIME: 50 TO 55 MINUTES

Pie doesn't have to be sweet to be delicious. This savory pie, filled with imitation crab and the Cajun trinity—onion, green bell pepper, and celery—is sure to become a favorite of any seafood lover. **SERVES 4**

- 1 (9-inch) gluten-free deep-dish piecrust, blind-baked
- 4 tablespoons (½ stick) salted butter, melted
- ½ cup chopped celery
- ½ cup chopped yellow onion
- 1 cup chopped green bell pepper
- 4 large eggs, beaten
- 1 cup whole milk
- 1 teaspoon sea salt
- ½ teaspoon cayenne pepper
- 1 cup shredded sharp Cheddar cheese
- 1 (8-ounce) package gluten-free imitation crab, (see ingredient tip)

1. Preheat the oven to 325°F.
2. In a medium skillet, combine the butter, celery, onion, and bell pepper. Sauté over medium heat for 5 to 7 minutes, or until the onion is tender and translucent. Remove from the heat.
3. In a medium bowl, whisk together the eggs, milk, salt, and cayenne until blended.
4. Stir in the cheese and imitation crab.
5. Spread the crab mixture evenly across the piecrust.
6. Transfer the piecrust to the oven, and bake for 40 to 45 minutes, or until a knife inserted into the center of the pie comes out clean. Remove from the oven. Let cool for 20 minutes.

STORAGE: Tightly wrap the pie in aluminum foil, or put in an airtight container. Refrigerate for up to 5 days, or freeze for up to 2 months.

THAWING AND REHEATING: Thaw in the refrigerator overnight. To reheat individual portions, wrap 1 slice in a damp paper towel. Microwave on 50 percent power for 1 minute.

INGREDIENT TIP: Imitation crab often contains wheat binders, so not all brands are gluten-free. Check the ingredient label before purchasing.

SUBSTITUTION TIP: Replace the imitation crab with 1 pound of crab or crawfish meat.

Per Serving: Calories: 661; Total fat: 44g; Saturated fat: 20g; Protein: 23g; Total carbs: 43g; Fiber: 2g; Sugar: 9g; Sodium: 1,262mg

Pepper Steak

PREP TIME: 20 MINUTES • COOK TIME: 25 TO 30 MINUTES

Quinoa replaces rice to give a new twist to an old favorite. Have any leftover pineapple juice from the Peach and Pineapple Smoothie (page 118)? It can be substituted for the water in this recipe. SERVES 4

1 tablespoon extra-virgin olive oil

1 yellow onion, chopped

1 green bell pepper, chopped

1 teaspoon sea salt

1 teaspoon garlic powder

1 teaspoon ground ginger

1 (14½-ounce) can diced tomatoes

1 pound boneless sirloin steak, cut into 1-inch-thick strips

1 tablespoon cornstarch

¼ cup water

3 tablespoons gluten-free soy sauce or tamari

1 tablespoon sugar

3 cups cooked quinoa

1. In a large saucepan, combine the oil, onion, and bell pepper. Cook over medium heat for 5 to 7 minutes, or until the onion is tender and translucent.

2. In a medium bowl, stir together the salt, garlic powder, ground ginger, and tomatoes with their juices until blended. Add to the saucepan, and stir to combine with the vegetables.

3. Add the steak, and stir until blended.

4. Reduce the heat to low. Cook, stirring occasionally, for 10 to 15 minutes, or until the steak is tender and brown.

5. To make a slurry, in a small bowl, whisk together the cornstarch, water, soy sauce, and sugar until blended.

6. Pour the slurry over the steak mixture, and cook for about 5 more minutes, stirring until thickened.

7. Stir in the quinoa. Remove from the heat. Let cool for 20 minutes.

STORAGE: Put in an airtight container. Refrigerate for up to 4 days, or freeze for up to 3 months.

THAWING AND REHEATING: Thaw in the refrigerator overnight. To reheat individual servings, put on a microwave-safe plate, and loosely cover with a paper towel. Microwave on 50 percent power for 1 minute. Stir and heat for 30 more seconds, if needed.

Per Serving: Calories: 476; Total fat: 19g; Saturated fat: 6g; Protein: 33g; Total carbs: 44g; Fiber: 7g; Sugar: 9g; Sodium: 1,526mg

Twice-Baked Potatoes

PREP TIME: 15 MINUTES • COOK TIME: 35 MINUTES

These fluffy stuffed potatoes overflow with cheese and herbs. A classic comfort food, these potatoes freeze well. Serve as a side or as a light meal. Microwaving the potatoes saves time and makes for easy preparation. SERVES 4

4 large Russet potatoes

Nonstick cooking spray, for coating the sheet pan

1 cup full-fat plain yogurt

¼ cup whole milk

1 teaspoon dried chives

½ teaspoon paprika

½ teaspoon garlic powder

½ teaspoon sea salt

½ teaspoon freshly ground black pepper

½ cup shredded sharp Cheddar cheese

2 bacon slices, cooked, drained, and crumbled (optional)

1. Using a fork, prick each potato 5 times on each side.

2. Put the potatoes in the microwave, and cook on high power for 16 minutes, flipping halfway through. Let cool for 10 minutes.

3. Preheat the oven to 350°F. Coat a sheet pan with cooking spray.

4. Halve the potatoes lengthwise. Scoop the flesh into a large bowl. Reserve the potato shells.

5. Add the yogurt, milk, chives, paprika, garlic powder, salt, and pepper. Using a handheld mixer, beat on medium speed for about 3 minutes, or until the mixture is smooth and creamy.

6. Turn off the mixer. Stir in the cheese.

7. Fill each potato shell with 1 cup of the mixture.

8. Place the potatoes in a single layer on the prepared sheet pan.

9. Transfer the sheet pan to the oven, and bake for 10 to 15 minutes, or until heated through. Remove from the oven.

10. Sprinkle with the bacon (if using). Let cool for 20 minutes.

STORAGE: Tightly wrap each potato in foil, or put in airtight containers. Refrigerate for up to 5 days, or freeze for up to 3 months.

CONTINUED ⟶

THAWING AND REHEATING: Thaw in the refrigerator overnight. To reheat, put a potato on a microwave-safe dish. Microwave on high power for 45 seconds. Stir the filling, and heat for 30 more seconds, if needed.

VARIATION TIP: If you like, during step 6, add 1 cup diced ham, 1 teaspoon dried minced onion, or ½ cup shredded Italian-blend cheese.

Per Serving: Calories: 398; Total fat: 8g; Saturated fat: 4g; Protein: 14g; Total carbs: 71g; Fiber: 4g; Sugar: 6g; Sodium: 435mg

Fruity Mixed Greens Salad

PREP TIME: 20 MINUTES

Oranges, strawberries, and bacon may seem like an unusual combination, but it works well in this fruity salad. Topped with a tart fruity dressing, this salad is a delicious lunch or light dinner. **SERVES 4**

For the salad

1 (11-ounce) can mandarin orange slices, drained

1 pound fresh strawberries, hulled and sliced

1 yellow onion, chopped

1 (1-pound) package mixed greens

10 bacon slices, cooked, drained, and crumbled

¼ cup crumbled goat cheese, divided

For the dressing

½ cup freshly squeezed orange juice

¼ cup extra-virgin olive oil

¼ cup distilled white vinegar

2 tablespoons sugar

To make the salad

1. Using a paper towel, pat the oranges and strawberries dry.

2. Put ⅓ cup of oranges in each of 4 (1-pint) Mason jars.

3. Top each jar of oranges with the following, in the order listed: ½ cup of strawberries, ¼ cup of onion, 1 cup of mixed greens, one-fourth of the bacon, and 1 tablespoon of goat cheese. To prepare 1 large salad, in a large bowl or on a serving platter, layer the ingredients as listed.

To make the dressing

4. In a small bowl, whisk together the orange juice, oil, vinegar, and sugar until the sugar has dissolved and the mixture has combined.

STORAGE: Refrigerate the salads for up to 5 days. Divide the dressing among 4 (1-ounce) containers, and refrigerate for up to 5 days. The salad should not be frozen.

SUBSTITUTION TIP: Replace the orange juice in the dressing with lemon or lime juice. Replace the mandarin orange slices with pineapple chunks.

Per Serving: Calories: 378; Total fat: 24g; Saturated fat: 6g; Protein: 12g; Total carbs: 30g; Fiber: 5g; Sugar: 23g; Sodium: 489mg

Peach and Pineapple Smoothie

PREP TIME: 15 MINUTES

This three-fruit smoothie will remind you of the warm, balmy breezes during a tropical vacation. Reserve and freeze any leftover peach and pineapple juice to use in smoothies, fruit dressings, or ice pops. SERVES 4

1 (15-ounce) can pineapple chunks in juice, strained, 1 cup juice reserved

1 (15-ounce) can sliced peaches in juice, drained

3 bananas, peeled, cut into thirds, and frozen

1 (1-pound) container full-fat vanilla yogurt

1. In a high-speed blender, combine the reserved pineapple juice, pineapple chunks, peaches, bananas, and yogurt. Pulse for 10 to 12 seconds, or until smooth.

2. To prepare individual servings, pour the smoothie into 4 (8-ounce) Mason jars. Seal the jars.

STORAGE: Refrigerate for up to 4 days, or freeze for up to 2 months.

THAWING AND REHEATING: Thaw in the refrigerator overnight. Stir before serving.

SUBSTITUTION TIP: One (16-ounce) package of frozen mixed fruit can replace the pineapple and peaches. Replace the vanilla yogurt with your favorite flavor.

- -

Per Serving: Calories: 252; Total fat: 4g; Saturated fat: 2g; Protein: 6g; Total carbs: 53g; Fiber: 4g; Sugar: 41g; Sodium: 58mg

Fruit, Seed, and Nut Trail Mix

PREP TIME: 5 MINUTES

The sweet and salty flavor of this trail mix shines through in every bite. Mixed nuts and dried fruit blend to deliver chewiness and crunchiness for a pleasing mouthfeel. **MAKES 5¼ CUPS**

1 (10½-ounce) container mixed nuts

1 (8-ounce) package sunflower seeds

1 (8-ounce) package pumpkin seeds

1 (1-pound) package dried mixed fruit

In a large bowl, combine the mixed nuts, sunflower seeds, pumpkin seeds, and dried fruit. Using clean hands, mix until blended.

STORAGE: Store in an airtight container at room temperature for up to 2 weeks, or freeze for up to 3 months.

THAWING AND REHEATING: Thaw at room temperature for 2 to 3 hours.

VARIATION TIP: Add 1 teaspoon cayenne pepper for a spicy version. Add 1 teaspoon ground cinnamon for a sweet version.

Per Serving (1 cup): Calories 1,224; Total fat: 91g; Saturated fat: 10g; Protein: 31g; Total carbs: 97g; Fiber: 19g; Sugar: 65g; Sodium: 15mg

FALL MENU:
Six-Recipe Meal Prep

The weather is cooling down, but it's heating up in the kitchen with these nourishing dishes. From a chunky vegetable soup to a shepherd's pie topped with fluffy mashed potatoes, you'll enjoy the taste and the simplicity of these meals. Lentils pack a protein power punch and add a twist to classic burritos. You won't miss the meat! The cookies freeze well, so feel free to double the recipe. They can also be baked to suit individual tastes: if you prefer a softer, chewier cookie, reduce the baking time by 2 minutes. Simple pantry swaps include semisweet or vanilla chips for milk chocolate chips, black beans for green beans, and rotini or penne noodles for elbow macaroni. Leftover ingredients, like extra cheese, can be used as a topping for the vegetable soup or mixed into the pancake batter before frying. Extra cooked lentils can be added to the shepherd's pie filling.

FALL MENU:
Six-Recipe Meal Prep Shopping List

PRODUCE
Apple, Granny Smith (1)
Avocado (1)
Bell pepper, green (1)
Carrots (2)
Celery (1 bunch)
Garlic (1 head)
Lemons (2)
Onions, yellow (3)
Potatoes, Russet (3)
Squash, yellow (2)

DAIRY AND EGGS
Butter, salted (8 ounces)
Buttermilk, low-fat (1 pint)
Cheese, Cheddar, sharp, shredded
   (1 [1-pound] bag)
Cheese, Italian-style, shredded
   (1 [8-ounce] bag)
Eggs, large (1 half dozen)
Milk, whole (1 pint)
Sour cream, full-fat (1 [8-ounce] container)

MEAT
Beef, ground, 80/20 (1 pound)
Sausage, pork (1 pound)

CANNED AND BOTTLED
Broth, vegetable (1 [32-ounce] container)
Corn, whole kernel (1 [15-ounce] can)
Green beans (2 [14½-ounce] cans)
Maple syrup (1 [8-ounce] bottle)
Olives, black, sliced (1 [15-ounce] jar)

Peanut butter, creamy (1 [1-pound] jar)
Salsa, mild, medium, or hot (1 [1-pound] jar)
Tomatoes, Italian-style, diced
   (1 [28-ounce] can)

PANTRY
Chocolate chips, milk chocolate
   (1 [11½-ounce] bag)
Elbow macaroni, gluten-free (1 [12-ounce]
   package)
Flour, all-purpose gluten-free one-to-one
   baking (1 [1-pound] package)
Lentils, brown or green (1 [1-pound]
   package)
Sugar, light brown (1 [1-pound] box)
Tortillas, flour, 8-inch, gluten-free
   (1 [8-count] package)
Vanilla extract (1 bottle)

CHECK YOUR PANTRY FOR . . .
Baking soda, black peppercorns,
cornstarch, dried mustard, extra-virgin
olive oil, garlic powder, gluten-free
hot pepper sauce, ground cumin,
Italian seasoning, nonstick cooking
spray, sea salt

Weekly Meal Chart

	BREAKFAST	LUNCH	DINNER	SNACK
DAY 1	Sausage and Apple Pancakes	Shepherd's Pie	Lentil Burritos	Peanut Butter–Chocolate Chip Cookies
DAY 2	Sausage and Apple Pancakes	Cheesy Macaroni Bake	Vegetable Soup	Peanut Butter–Chocolate Chip Cookies
DAY 3		Cheesy Macaroni Bake	Lentil Burritos	Peanut Butter–Chocolate Chip Cookies
DAY 4	Sausage and Apple Pancakes	Vegetable Soup	Shepherd's Pie	Peanut Butter–Chocolate Chip Cookies
DAY 5	Sausage and Apple Pancakes	Lentil Burritos	Cheesy Macaroni Bake	Peanut Butter–Chocolate Chip Cookies
DAY 6		Shepherd's Pie	Vegetable Soup	Peanut Butter–Chocolate Chip Cookies

STEP-BY-STEP PREP

1. Using a fork, prick 3 Russet potatoes 5 times on each side. Put the potatoes on a microwave-safe dish, and microwave on high for 10 minutes, flipping halfway through. Let cool for 10 minutes. Peel and dice.

2. Prep the vegetables for the week:

   ☐ *Juice enough lemons to measure 2 tablespoons juice.*

   ☐ *Core and chop enough of 1 Granny Smith apple to measure 1 cup, and sprinkle with the lemon juice.*

- ☐ *Seed and dice 1 green bell pepper.*

- ☐ *Thinly slice 2 yellow squash.*

- ☐ *Peel and thinly slice 2 carrots.*

- ☐ *Thinly slice 2 celery stalks.*

- ☐ *Dice 3 yellow onions, and divide into 3 (1-cup) portions.*

- ☐ *Mince enough garlic to measure 2 tablespoons.*

3. Cook the lentils. Rinse 1⅔ cups brown lentils in a strainer. In a large saucepan, combine the lentils and 5 cups water. Bring to a boil over high heat. Reduce the heat to low. Cover the pan, and simmer for 18 to 20 minutes, or until tender. Remove from the heat. Let sit for 5 minutes before using. Drain any excess water from the lentils. Wash the saucepan.

4. Cook the sausage. In a medium skillet, cook 1 pound pork sausage over medium heat, stirring to break up the meat, for 7 to 10 minutes, or until browned and no pink remains. Remove from the heat. Drain the sausage.

5. In the same saucepan used to cook the lentils, cook 12 ounces macaroni for 4 minutes less than the package directions indicate. Remove from the heat. Drain, and rinse with cool water.

6. Prepare the Shepherd's Pie (page 126) as directed. Let cool for 20 minutes. Put in an airtight container. Refrigerate for up to 4 days, or freeze for up to 3 months.

7. Prepare the Cheesy Macaroni Bake (page 128) as directed. Let cool for 20 minutes. Put in an airtight container. Refrigerate for up to 1 week, or freeze for up to 3 months.

8. Prepare the Vegetable Soup (page 129) as directed. Let cool for 20 minutes. Put in an airtight container, and refrigerate for up to 5 days, or freeze for up to 3 months. Divide ½ cup Italian-style cheese among 4 (1-ounce) containers (if using). Refrigerate for up to 1 week, or freeze for up to 3 months.

9. Prepare the Sausage and Apple Pancakes (page 130) as directed. Let cool for 10 minutes. Place a sheet of wax paper or parchment paper between each pancake, and put in a gallon-size freezer bag. Refrigerate for up to 5 days, or freeze for up to 2 months.

Divide ½ cup maple syrup among 4 (1-ounce) containers. Refrigerate for up to 1 year.

10. Prepare the Lentil Burritos (page 132) as directed. Let cool for 10 minutes. Tightly wrap each burrito in aluminum foil, or put in an airtight container. Refrigerate for up to 6 days, or freeze for up to 3 months. Divide ¼ cup sour cream among 4 (1-ounce) containers. Refrigerate for up to 1 week. The avocado should be prepped immediately before serving.

11. Prepare the Peanut Butter–Chocolate Chip Cookies (page 133) as directed. Let cool for 10 minutes. Store in an airtight container at room temperature for up to 5 days, or freeze for up to 3 months.

Shepherd's Pie

PREP TIME: 30 MINUTES • COOK TIME: 30 MINUTES

Originating in Scotland and later embraced in France as "hachis Parmentier," this dish once used lamb and a savory gravy. The newer versions, like this one, feature browned hamburger, tender onion, and a creamy, cheesy mashed potato topping. SERVES 4

For the pie

Nonstick cooking spray, for coating the baking dish

1 pound 80/20 ground beef

1 cup diced yellow onion

1 (14½-ounce) can green beans, drained

1 (14½-ounce) can Italian-style diced tomatoes, drained

1 (15-ounce) can whole kernel corn, drained

1 teaspoon Italian seasoning

1 teaspoon garlic powder

1 teaspoon sea salt

½ teaspoon freshly ground black pepper

1 tablespoon cornstarch

1 tablespoon water

For the topping

3 diced, peeled, cooked Russet potatoes

½ cup whole milk

1 large egg, beaten

1 cup shredded sharp Cheddar cheese

To make the pie

1. Preheat the oven to 350°F. Coat a 9-by-13-inch baking dish with cooking spray.

2. In a medium skillet, combine the beef and onion. Cook over medium heat for 7 to 10 minutes, or until the beef has browned and no pink remains. Remove from the heat. Drain.

3. In a large bowl, stir together the green beans, tomatoes, corn, Italian seasoning, garlic powder, salt, and pepper until combined.

4. Add the beef and onion mixture.

5. To make a slurry, in a small bowl, whisk together the cornstarch and water until blended.

6. Stir the slurry into the ground beef mixture.

7. Spread the beef mixture into the prepared baking dish.

To make the topping

8. In a large bowl, combine the potatoes, milk, egg, and cheese. Using a handheld mixer, mix on low speed for about 5 minutes, or until the potatoes are fluffy.

9. Spread the potato mixture evenly over the beef mixture.

10. Transfer the baking dish to the oven, and bake for 30 minutes, or until the potatoes are set. Remove from the oven. Let cool for 20 minutes.

STORAGE: Put in an airtight container. Refrigerate for up to 4 days, or freeze for up to 3 months.

THAWING AND REHEATING: Thaw in the refrigerator overnight. To reheat individual servings, put in a microwave-safe dish. Microwave on high power for 45 seconds. Heat for 30 more seconds, if needed.

SUBSTITUTION TIP: In a hurry? Use 1 (4-ounce) package instant Cheddar-flavored mashed potatoes, prepared as directed on the package, to replace the potato topping.

- -

Per Serving: Calories: 647; Total fat: 36g; Saturated fat: 15g; Protein: 35g; Total carbs: 48g; Fiber: 8g; Sugar: 9g; Sodium: 960mg

Cheesy Macaroni Bake

PREP TIME: 20 MINUTES • COOK TIME: 20 MINUTES

A rich, gooey blend of cheeses gives this classic baked dish new life. Although this recipe does require a bit of prep time, each forkful of these tender noodles is worth the effort. **SERVES 4**

Nonstick cooking spray, for coating the baking dish

1 tablespoon salted butter

¼ cup all-purpose gluten-free one-to-one baking flour

1 cup whole milk

1 cup shredded Italian-style cheese

½ cup shredded sharp Cheddar cheese

¼ cup full-fat sour cream

1 teaspoon dried mustard

1 teaspoon sea salt

1 teaspoon freshly ground black pepper

1 (12-ounce) package gluten-free elbow macaroni, cooked for 4 minutes less than the package directions indicate

1. Preheat the oven to 350°F. Coat a 9-by-9-inch baking dish with cooking spray.

2. In a large skillet, melt the butter over medium heat.

3. Stir in the flour until blended.

4. Slowly add the milk, stirring constantly, until the flour has dissolved.

5. Add the Italian-style cheese, Cheddar cheese, sour cream, mustard, salt, and pepper. Cook, stirring, for 3 to 5 minutes, or until the mixture is smooth and the cheese has melted.

6. Stir in the macaroni. Remove from the heat.

7. Pour the macaroni mixture into the prepared baking dish.

8. Transfer the baking dish to the oven, and bake for 20 minutes, or until set. Remove from the oven. Let cool for 20 minutes.

STORAGE: Put in an airtight container. Refrigerate for up to 1 week, or freeze for up to 3 months.

THAWING AND REHEATING: Thaw in the refrigerator overnight. To heat individual servings, put on a microwave-safe plate. Microwave on high power for 45 seconds. Stir and heat for 30 more seconds, if needed.

Per Serving: Calories: 602; Total fat: 24g; Saturated fat: 14g; Protein: 19g; Total carbs: 76g; Fiber: 3g; Sugar: 4g; Sodium: 924mg

Vegetable Soup

PREP TIME: 15 MINUTES • COOK TIME: 35 TO 40 MINUTES

Six vegetables combine in this broth-based soup. Canned vegetables and seasoned tomatoes make this a convenient recipe for last-minute meals. Any leftover Italian-style cheese can be used as a topping. SERVES 4

2 tablespoons extra-virgin olive oil

1 cup diced yellow onion

2 carrots, thinly sliced

2 celery stalks, thinly sliced

4 cups vegetable broth

1 teaspoon sea salt

1 teaspoon freshly ground black pepper

1 teaspoon Italian seasoning

1 (14½-ounce) can Italian-style diced tomatoes

1 (14½-ounce) can green beans, drained

2 yellow squash, thinly sliced

1 tablespoon cornstarch

1 tablespoon water

½ cup shredded Italian-style cheese (optional)

1. In a large saucepan, combine the oil, onion, carrots, and celery. Sauté over medium heat for 5 to 7 minutes, or until the onion is tender and translucent.

2. Stir in the broth, salt, pepper, Italian seasoning, and tomatoes with their juices. Bring to a boil.

3. Add the green beans and squash. Cover the pan.

4. Reduce the heat to low. Simmer, stirring occasionally, for 15 to 20 minutes, or until the squash is fork-tender.

5. To make a slurry, in a small bowl, whisk together the cornstarch and water until blended.

6. Stir the slurry into the soup. Simmer for 5 more minutes, or until thickened slightly. Remove from the heat. Let cool for 20 minutes.

7. Serve the soup with the cheese (if using).

STORAGE: Put in an airtight container. Refrigerate for up to 5 days, or freeze for up to 3 months. Divide the cheese among 4 (1-ounce) containers (if using). Refrigerate for up to 1 week, or freeze for up to 3 months.

THAWING AND REHEATING: Thaw in the refrigerator overnight. To reheat individual servings, put in a microwave-safe bowl. Heat on high power for 30 seconds. Stir and heat for 30 seconds to 1 minute more, or until warm. Stir before serving, and top with cheese.

Per Serving: Calories: 153; Total fat: 8g; Saturated fat: 1g; Protein: 4g; Total carbs: 20g; Fiber: 7g; Sugar: 9g; Sodium: 635mg

Sausage and Apple Pancakes

PREP TIME: 20 MINUTES • COOK TIME: 20 MINUTES

Savory pancakes topped with a pat of butter and syrup make for an unbeatable breakfast. Use your choice of hot or mild sausage to adjust the heat level of these pancakes. SERVES 4

1 cup chopped Granny
    Smith apple

2 tablespoons freshly
    squeezed lemon juice

1⅔ cups all-purpose
    gluten-free one-to-one
    baking flour

½ teaspoon sea salt

1 teaspoon baking soda

2 large eggs, beaten

2 cups low-fat buttermilk

1 pound pork sausage,
    cooked and crumbled

Nonstick cooking spray, for
    coating the skillet

½ cup maple syrup

1. In a small bowl, coat the apple with the lemon juice to prevent browning.

2. In another small bowl, stir together the flour, salt, and baking soda.

3. In a large bowl, whisk together the eggs and buttermilk until blended.

4. To make the batter, add the flour mixture to the egg mixture, and whisk until blended. The batter will be lumpy.

5. Add the apple and the sausage. Stir to blend.

6. Coat a medium skillet with cooking spray, and heat over medium heat.

7. Make 1 pancake at a time by adding ¾ cup of the batter to the skillet. Cook for 2 to 3 minutes. Flip, and cook for 1 to 2 minutes, or until set. Transfer to a plate. Continue with the remaining batter, coating the skillet with cooking spray before each pancake. This should make 4 large pancakes. Turn off the heat. Let cool for 10 minutes.

8. Serve the pancakes with the syrup.

STORAGE: Place a sheet of wax or parchment paper between each pancake, and put in a gallon-size freezer bag. Refrigerate for up to 5 days, or freeze for up to 2 months. Divide the syrup among 4 (1-ounce) containers. Refrigerate for up to 1 year.

THAWING AND REHEATING: Thaw in the refrigerator overnight, or reheat from frozen. To reheat individual servings, put a frozen pancake on a microwave-safe plate. Microwave on high power for 1 to 1½ minutes. Thawed pancakes can be reheated for 30 seconds.

VARIATION TIP: Any type of cooking apple can be used here—Jonagold, winesap, or Pink Lady is also a good choice.

Per Serving: Calories: 807; Total fat: 41g; Saturated fat: 15g; Protein: 30g; Total carbs: 78g; Fiber: 2g; Sugar: 33g; Sodium: 1,404mg

Lentil Burritos

PREP TIME: 15 MINUTES • COOK TIME: 20 MINUTES

Tired of bean burritos? Easy-to-cook lentils add the firm texture of beans, along with a nutty flavor. Filled with salsa, cheese, and other goodies, this recipe will become a staple for burrito lovers. **SERVES 4**

2 tablespoons extra-virgin olive oil

1 cup diced yellow onion

1 green bell pepper, seeded and diced

2 tablespoons minced garlic

4 cups cooked brown or green lentils

1 (16-ounce) jar mild, medium, or hot salsa

1 tablespoon gluten-free hot pepper sauce

1 teaspoon ground cumin

1 (15-ounce) can sliced black olives, drained

8 (8-inch) gluten-free flour tortillas

1 cup shredded sharp Cheddar cheese

¼ cup full-fat sour cream

1 ripe avocado, pitted, peeled, and sliced

1. In a large skillet, combine the oil, onion, bell pepper, and garlic. Sauté over medium heat, stirring often, for 5 to 7 minutes, or until the onion is tender and translucent.

2. Stir in the lentils, salsa, hot sauce, and cumin. Bring to a boil.

3. Reduce the heat to low. Cover the skillet, and simmer for 10 minutes. Remove from the heat.

4. Stir in the olives.

5. Spread 1 cup of the lentil mixture evenly down the center of each tortilla.

6. Top each with 2 tablespoons of cheese.

7. Fold the tortillas burrito-style. Let cool for 10 minutes.

8. Serve the burritos with the sour cream and avocado.

STORAGE: Tightly wrap each burrito in aluminum foil, or put in an airtight container. Refrigerate for up to 6 days, or freeze for up to 3 months. Divide the sour cream among 4 (1-ounce) containers. Refrigerate for up to 1 week. The avocado should be prepped immediately before serving.

THAWING AND REHEATING: Thaw in the refrigerator overnight. To reheat individual servings, put a burrito on a microwave-safe plate. Microwave on high power for 45 seconds. Flip and heat for 30 more seconds, if needed.

Per Serving: Calories: 1,003; Total fat: 49g; Saturated fat: 15g; Protein: 36g; Total carbs: 116g; Fiber: 36g; Sugar: 19g; Sodium: 2,240mg

Peanut Butter-Chocolate Chip Cookies

PREP TIME: 10 MINUTES • COOK TIME: 10 TO 15 MINUTES

The flavors of chocolate and peanut butter come through in every bite of these chewy cookies. Feel free to add extra chocolate chips, or if you have a peanut allergy, use almond butter or cashew butter instead. **MAKES 10 COOKIES**

Nonstick cooking spray, for coating the sheet pan

1 cup creamy peanut butter

1 cup packed light brown sugar

1 large egg, beaten

1 teaspoon vanilla extract

½ cup milk chocolate chips

1. Preheat the oven to 325°F. Coat a sheet pan with cooking spray.

2. To make the dough, in a medium bowl, combine the peanut butter, sugar, and egg. Using a handheld mixer, beat on medium speed for 2 to 3 minutes, or until blended.

3. Turn off the mixer. Add the vanilla and chocolate chips. Stir until combined.

4. Divide the dough into 10 portions, and roll each into a ball.

5. Put the balls on the prepared sheet pan, and flatten each using a fork.

6. Transfer the sheet pan to the oven, and bake for 10 to 12 minutes, or until browned. Remove from the oven. Let cool for 10 minutes.

STORAGE: Put in an airtight container. Store at room temperature for up to 5 days, or freeze for up to 3 months.

THAWING AND REHEATING: Let sit at room temperature for 20 to 30 minutes.

PREPARATION TIP: Know your sheet pans. Light-colored sheet pans reflect heat. Use them to reduce the risk of burning the cookies. Dark sheet pans absorb heat, causing baked goods to brown faster. If using a dark pan, reduce the cooking time to 8 to 10 minutes.

Per Serving: Calories: 287; Total fat: 16g; Saturated fat: 4g; Protein: 7g; Total carbs: 32g; Fiber: 2g; Sugar: 27g; Sodium: 120mg

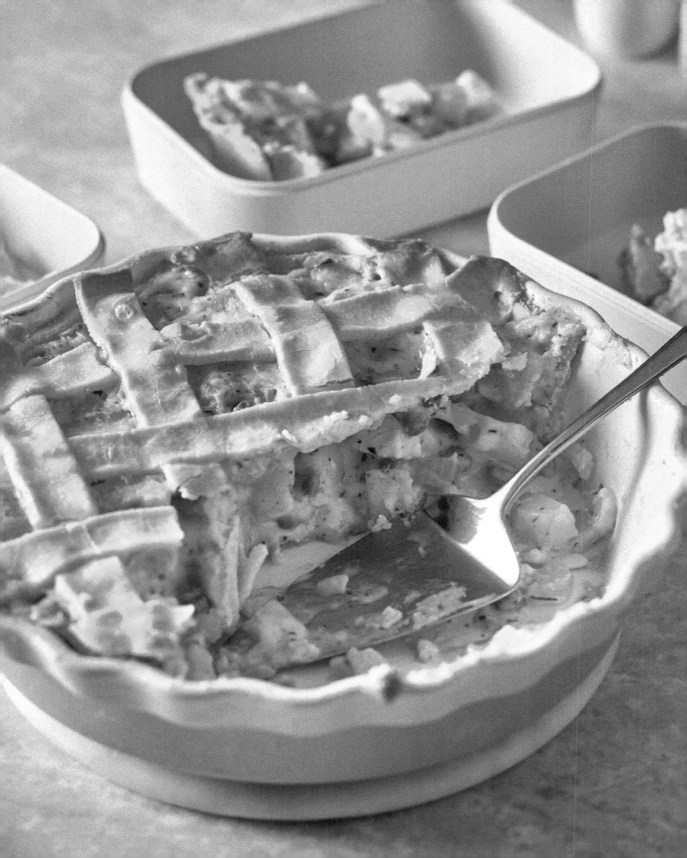

WINTER MENU:
Six-Recipe Meal Prep

There's nothing like the comfort of a home-cooked meal when frigid temperatures, biting winds, and snow drive us indoors. This prep brings a variety of new flavors with a steamy soup, a creamy potpie studded with vegetables, and "meatballs" with a lightly spiced pumpkin sauce. We'll finish the meals with a chewy blondie. Pantry swaps include pecans for walnuts and dark brown sugar for light. If you have unsalted butter in the refrigerator, use it instead of salted butter. Chicken broth and vegetable broth can be used interchangeably in the pumpkin sauce and potpie. Leftover bacon, cheese, and chives make for tasty toppings for the soup or the pumpkin sauce. Leftover eggs can be fried and used as an additional topping on the oatmeal. If you prefer not to add wine to your recipes, simply replace it with an equal amount of vegetable broth.

‹‹ Chicken Potpie, page 141

WINTER MENU:
Six-Recipe Meal Prep Shopping List

PRODUCE
Bell peppers, green (2)
Celery (1 bunch)
Chives (2 bunches)
Eggplant (1)
Garlic (1 head)
Lemons (2)
Onions, yellow (3)
Potato, Russet (1)

DAIRY AND EGGS
Butter, salted (1 pound)
Cheese, Italian-style, shredded
  (1 [8-ounce] bag)
Eggs, large (1 half dozen)
Milk, whole (1 quart)

MEAT
Bacon (1 [12-ounce] package)
Beef, ground, 80/20 (1 pound)
Chicken, breast, boneless, skinless
  (8 ounces)

FROZEN FOOD
Peas and carrots (1 [10-ounce] package)
Piecrust, gluten-free, deep dish, 9-inch (2)

CANNED AND BOTTLED
Broth, chicken (1 [14½-ounce] can)
Broth, vegetable (1 [14½-ounce] can)

Lentils (1 [15-ounce] can)
Pumpkin (1 [15-ounce] can)
Tomatoes, diced (1 [28-ounce] can)
Tomato sauce (1 [14½-ounce] can)

PANTRY
Bread, gluten-free (1 loaf)
Flour, all-purpose gluten-free one-to-one
  baking (1 [1-pound] package)
Sugar, light brown (1 [1-pound] package)
Oats, gluten-free, old-fashioned
  (1 [2-pound] package)
Pasta, gluten-free (1 [12-ounce] package)
Walnuts, chopped (1 cup)

OTHER
Wine, white (1 [750-mL] bottle; optional)

CHECK YOUR PANTRY FOR . . .
Black peppercorns, chili powder,
dried basil, dried marjoram, dried
oregano, dried parsley, dried rosemary, dried sage, dried thyme,
extra-virgin olive oil, garlic powder,
ground nutmeg, Italian seasoning,
nonstick cooking spray, sea salt,
vanilla extract

Weekly Meal Chart

	BREAKFAST	LUNCH	DINNER	SNACK
DAY 1	Bacon and Chive Oatmeal	Lentil Soup	Beef and Eggplant Casserole	Walnut Blondies
DAY 2	Bacon and Chive Oatmeal	Chicken Potpie	Oatmeal "Meatballs" with Pumpkin Sauce	Walnut Blondies
DAY 3		Beef and Eggplant Casserole	Lentil Soup	Walnut Blondies
DAY 4	Bacon and Chive Oatmeal	Oatmeal "Meatballs" with Pumpkin Sauce	Chicken Potpie	Walnut Blondies
DAY 5	Bacon and Chive Oatmeal	Lentil Soup	Beef and Eggplant Casserole	Walnut Blondies
DAY 6		Oatmeal "Meatballs" with Pumpkin Sauce	Chicken Potpie	Walnut Blondies

STEP-BY-STEP PREP

1. Prep the vegetables for the week:

   ☐ *Dice enough Russet potato to measure 1 cup.*

   ☐ *Dice 1 eggplant.*

   ☐ *Chop 2 yellow onions, and set aside. Chop enough of the remaining onion to measure ½ cup, and dice enough to measure ½ cup.*

   ☐ *Seed and chop 2 green bell peppers.*

☐ *Chop enough chives to measure 1 cup (¼ cup is optional).*

☐ *Dice enough celery to measure 1 (⅓-cup) and 1 (¼-cup) portion.*

☐ *Mince enough garlic to measure 3 tablespoons.*

☐ *Juice enough lemons to measure 2 tablespoons juice.*

2. Cook the chicken. In a large saucepan, combine 8 ounces boneless, skinless chicken breasts and 2 cups water. Bring to a boil over medium heat. Reduce the heat to medium-low. Cook for 10 to 15 minutes, or until the chicken reaches an internal temperature of 165°F. Remove from the heat. Transfer the chicken to a cutting board. Once cool enough to handle, dice. Wash the pan.

3. Cook the ground beef. In a medium skillet, cook 1 pound ground beef over medium heat, stirring to break up the beef, for 7 to 10 minutes, or until browned and no pink remains. Remove from the heat. Drain the beef. Wipe out the skillet.

4. Cook the bacon. In the same skillet, cook 12 bacon slices (or just 10, if omitting from the Lentil Soup) over medium heat, turning every 2 to 3 minutes, for 7 to 10 minutes, or until they reach your desired crispness. Remove from the heat. Transfer to paper towels to drain and cool. Crumble the bacon.

5. In the saucepan used to cook the chicken, cook 12 ounces pasta for 4 minutes less than the package directions indicate. Remove from the heat. Drain, and rinse with cool water.

6. Preheat the oven to 350°F.

7. Blind-bake 1 piecrust. Using a fork, prick holes in the bottom and sides. Put the piecrust in the oven, and bake for 10 minutes, or until lightly browned. Remove from the oven.

8. Cook the Beef and Eggplant Casserole (page 140) as directed. Let cool for 25 minutes. Put in an airtight container. Refrigerate for up to 3 days, or freeze for up to 3 months.

9. Place the remaining piecrust on the counter to thaw for 10 to 15 minutes while you cook the Chicken Potpie (page 141) as directed (the crust will be thawed sufficiently to cut it into strips for topping the pie). Let the potpie cool for 25 minutes. Tightly wrap

in aluminum foil. Refrigerate for up to 3 days, or freeze for up to 3 months.

10. Cook the Walnut Blondies (page 143) as directed. Let cool for 20 minutes. Put in an air-tight container, adding 1 piece of gluten-free bread on top to keep the blondies soft. Store at room temperature for up to 5 days, refrigerate for 1 week, or freeze for up to 3 months.

11. Cook the Lentil Soup (page 144) as directed. Let cool for 20 minutes. Put in an airtight container. Refrig-erate for up to 5 days, or freeze for up to 3 months. In each of 4 (2-ounce) containers, combine

1 tablespoon Italian-style cheese (if using), 1 tablespoon chives (if using), and one-fourth of the bacon (if using). Refrigerate for up to 4 days.

12. Cook the Oatmeal "Meatballs" with Pumpkin Sauce (page 145) as directed. Let cool for 15 minutes. Put in an airtight container. Refrig-erate for up to 5 days, or freeze for up to 3 months.

13. Cook the Bacon and Chive Oat-meal (page 147) as directed. Let cool for 10 minutes. Put in an airtight container. Refrigerate for up to 5 days, or freeze for up to 3 months.

Beef and Eggplant Casserole

PREP TIME: 20 MINUTES • COOK TIME: 45 TO 50 MINUTES

Casseroles are known for being catchall dishes for cleaning out the refrigerator. Not this one! Chunky eggplant, a blend of cheeses, and a seasoned tomato sauce will have you clamoring for more. **SERVES 4**

Nonstick cooking spray, for coating the baking dish

2 tablespoons extra-virgin olive oil

1 yellow onion, chopped

1 green bell pepper, seeded and chopped

1 (14½-ounce) can tomato sauce

1 teaspoon sea salt

1 teaspoon dried oregano

1 teaspoon dried basil

1 teaspoon Italian seasoning

½ teaspoon freshly ground black pepper

1 pound 80/20 ground beef, cooked and drained

1 eggplant, diced

1 cup shredded Italian-style cheese

1. Preheat the oven to 350°F. Coat a 9-by-13-inch baking dish with cooking spray.

2. In a large skillet, combine the oil, onion, and bell pepper. Cook over medium heat for 5 to 7 minutes, or until the onion is tender and translucent.

3. Stir in the tomato sauce, salt, oregano, basil, Italian seasoning, pepper, and beef.

4. Reduce the heat to low. Simmer, stirring occasionally, for 10 minutes, or until the sauce has thickened. Remove from the heat.

5. Arrange the eggplant in the prepared baking dish, spreading it evenly.

6. Cover the eggplant with the meat sauce.

7. Transfer the baking dish to the oven, and bake for 20 to 25 minutes, or until the eggplant is fork-tender.

8. Evenly sprinkle the cheese over the casserole. Bake for 5 more minutes, or until the cheese has melted. Remove from the oven. Let cool for 25 minutes.

STORAGE: Put in an airtight container. Refrigerate for up to 3 days, or freeze for up to 3 months.

THAWING AND REHEATING: Thaw in the refrigerator overnight. To reheat individual servings, put on a microwave-safe dish. Microwave on high power for 45 seconds. Stir and heat for 30 more seconds.

Per Serving: Calories: 545; Total fat: 39g; Saturated fat: 15g; Protein: 30g; Total carbs: 22g; Fiber: 7g; Sugar: 12g; Sodium: 860mg

Chicken Potpie

PREP TIME: 20 MINUTES • COOK TIME: 45 MINUTES

A gluten-free diet doesn't mean you have to give up comfort foods. Bursting with chicken and an herbal, creamy sauce, this recipe uses two gluten-free piecrusts to speed up preparation time. **SERVES 4**

For poultry seasoning mix

1 teaspoon dried thyme

½ teaspoon dried rosemary

½ teaspoon dried marjoram

½ teaspoon freshly ground black pepper

¼ teaspoon ground nutmeg

For the potpie

1 cup diced Russet potato

½ cup diced yellow onion

⅓ cup diced celery

½ cup frozen peas and carrots

8 ounces boneless, skinless chicken breasts, cooked and diced

1 teaspoon sea salt

1 teaspoon freshly ground black pepper

4 tablespoons (½ stick) salted butter, melted

¼ cup all-purpose gluten-free one-to-one baking flour

1 cup chicken broth

½ cup whole milk

1 (9-inch) gluten-free deep-dish frozen piecrust, blind-baked

To make the seasoning mix

1. In a small bowl, stir together the thyme, rosemary, marjoram, pepper, and nutmeg until blended.

To make the potpie

2. Preheat the oven to 375°F.

3. In a large bowl, stir together the potato, onion, celery, peas and carrots, and chicken.

4. Add the seasoning mix, salt, and pepper. Using clean hands, mix until blended.

5. In a medium bowl, whisk together the butter and flour until the flour has dissolved.

6. To make a slurry, add the broth and milk to the medium bowl. Whisk until smooth and combined.

7. Stir the slurry into the chicken mixture until blended.

8. Put the blind-baked piecrust on a sheet pan. Spoon the chicken mixture into the piecrust.

9. Put the unbaked piecrust on a piece of wax paper. Cut the piecrust into 1-inch strips.

10. Place 4 strips horizontally across the chicken mixture. Top with 4 strips placed vertically. Cover with aluminum foil.

11. Transfer the sheet pan to the oven and bake for 35 minutes.

CONTINUED ⟶

1 (9-inch) gluten-free deep-dish frozen piecrust, thawed at room temperature for 10 to 15 minutes

12. Remove the foil. Bake for 10 minutes, or until the crust has lightly browned. Remove from the oven. Let cool for 25 minutes.

STORAGE: Tightly wrap the pie in aluminum foil. Refrigerate for up to 3 days, or freeze for up to 3 months.

THAWING AND REHEATING: Thaw in the refrigerator overnight. To reheat individual servings, put on a microwave-safe plate. Microwave on high power for 45 seconds. Heat for 30 more seconds, if needed.

Per Serving: Calories: 787; Total fat: 46g; Saturated fat: 17g; Protein: 22g; Total carbs: 71g; Fiber: 4g; Sugar: 3g; Sodium: 1,135mg

Walnut Blondies

PREP TIME: 15 MINUTES • COOK TIME: 25 MINUTES

You'll go nuts for these blondies. Loaded with walnuts in almost every bite, they are ready to pop in the oven in about 15 minutes. Brown sugar lends a hint of toffee and caramel flavor. **SERVES 6**

Nonstick cooking spray, for coating the baking dish

12 tablespoons (1½ sticks) salted butter, melted

2 cups packed light brown sugar

3 large eggs, beaten

1 teaspoon vanilla extract

1½ cups all-purpose gluten-free one-to-one baking flour

1 cup chopped walnuts

1. Preheat the oven to 350°F. Line a 9-by-13-inch baking dish with parchment paper, and coat with cooking spray.

2. In a large bowl, using a handheld mixer, cream the butter and sugar on medium speed for about 3 minutes, or until light and fluffy.

3. Add the eggs and vanilla. Mix until blended.

4. To make the batter, add the flour, and mix until well blended.

5. Turn off the mixer. Stir in the walnuts.

6. Pour the batter into the prepared baking dish.

7. Transfer the baking dish to the oven, and bake for 20 to 25 minutes, or until a knife inserted into the middle of the batter comes out clean. Remove from the oven. Let cool for 20 minutes.

STORAGE: Put in an airtight container, adding 1 piece gluten-free bread on top to keep the blondies soft. Store at room temperature for up to 5 days, refrigerate for 1 week, or freeze for up to 3 months.

THAWING AND REHEATING: Thaw at room temperature for 2 hours.

VARIATION TIP: Make triple chocolate–walnut brownies. Add 2 tablespoons unsweetened cocoa powder when adding the eggs and vanilla. Stir in ½ cup milk chocolate chips and ½ cup white chocolate chips with the walnuts.

Per Serving: Calories: 1,143; Total fat: 58g; Saturated fat: 24g; Protein: 15g; Total carbs: 148g; Fiber: 3g; Sugar: 108g; Sodium: 360mg

Lentil Soup

PREP TIME: 20 MINUTES • COOK TIME: 30 MINUTES

Canned lentils are the time-saving secret behind this speedy soup. This soup freezes well so feel free to make an extra batch. Any leftover diced potato can be added with the tomatoes, if you like. SERVES 4

¼ cup extra-virgin olive oil

1 yellow onion, chopped

1 green bell pepper, seeded and chopped

¼ cup diced celery

1 tablespoon minced garlic

1 (28-ounce) can diced tomatoes

½ cup white wine or vegetable broth

½ teaspoon sea salt

½ teaspoon freshly ground black pepper

½ teaspoon dried basil

½ teaspoon dried oregano

1 tablespoon dried parsley

2 tablespoons freshly squeezed lemon juice

1 (15-ounce) can lentils, drained and rinsed

¾ cup frozen peas and carrots

¼ cup shredded Italian-style cheese (optional)

¼ cup chopped fresh chives (optional)

2 bacon slices, cooked, drained, and crumbled (optional)

1. In a large saucepan, combine the oil, onion, bell pepper, celery, and garlic. Cook over medium heat for 5 to 7 minutes, or until the onion is tender and transparent.

2. Add the tomatoes with their juices, wine, salt, pepper, basil, oregano, parsley, and lemon juice. Bring to a boil.

3. Reduce the heat to low. Cover the pan, and simmer, stirring occasionally, for 15 minutes, or until the soup has thickened.

4. Add the lentils and peas and carrots. Cover the pan, and cook for 5 minutes. Remove from the heat. Let cool for 20 minutes.

5. Serve the soup with the cheese (if using), chives (if using), and bacon (if using).

STORAGE: Put in an airtight container. Refrigerate for up to 5 days, or freeze for up to 3 months. In each of 4 (2-ounce) containers, combine 1 tablespoon cheese (if using), 1 tablespoon chives (if using), and one-fourth of the bacon (if using). Refrigerate for up to 4 days.

THAWING AND REHEATING: Thaw in the refrigerator overnight. To reheat individual servings, put the soup in a microwave-safe bowl, and loosely cover with a paper towel. Microwave on 50 percent power for 1 minute. Stir and heat for 30 more seconds, if needed. Stir before serving, then top with the garnishes (if using).

Per Serving: Calories: 275; Total fat: 15g; Saturated fat: 2g; Protein: 10g; Total carbs: 30g; Fiber: 12g; Sugar: 9g; Sodium: 550mg

Oatmeal "Meatballs" with Pumpkin Sauce

PREP TIME: 15 MINUTES • COOK TIME: 20 TO 25 MINUTES

A savory pumpkin sauce and cheese and herb oatmeal "meatballs" create a surprising new take on a traditional spaghetti and meatball dinner. For even more pumpkin goodness, top with Cajun-Spiced Pumpkin Seeds (page 188). SERVES 4

For the "meatballs"

2 pieces gluten-free bread

1 cup gluten-free old-fashioned oats

¾ cup shredded Italian-style cheese

½ cup chopped yellow onion

3 large eggs, beaten

1 teaspoon dried parsley

1 teaspoon dried sage

½ teaspoon garlic powder

½ teaspoon sea salt

For the sauce

1 tablespoon salted butter

2 tablespoons minced garlic

1 cup canned pumpkin

1 cup vegetable broth

¼ cup whole milk

1 teaspoon freshly ground black pepper

½ teaspoon sea salt

½ teaspoon chili powder

1 (12-ounce) package gluten-free pasta, cooked for 4 minutes less than the package directions indicate

To make the "meatballs"

1. In a food processor or blender, process the bread for 5 to 10 seconds to make fine crumbs.

2. In a large bowl, combine the oats, cheese, onion, eggs, parsley, sage, garlic powder, salt, and bread crumbs. Using clean hands, mix until blended. Shape into 1-inch balls.

To make the sauce

3. In a large skillet, melt the butter over medium heat.

4. Add the "meatballs," and cook, stirring often, for 5 minutes, or until browned.

5. Add the garlic. Cook, stirring constantly, for 1 to 2 minutes, or until the garlic has lightly browned.

6. In a medium bowl, whisk together the pumpkin, broth, milk, pepper, salt, and chili powder until blended. Add to the skillet.

7. Reduce the heat to low. Simmer for 15 minutes, or until the sauce has slightly thickened.

8. Stir in the pasta until coated. Remove from the heat. Let cool for 15 minutes.

STORAGE: Put in an airtight container. Refrigerate for up to 5 days, or freeze for up to 3 months.

CONTINUED ⟶

THAWING AND REHEATING: Thaw in the refrigerator overnight. To reheat individual servings, put in a microwave-safe bowl, and cover with a paper towel. Microwave on high power for 30 seconds. Stir and heat for 30 more seconds, if needed.

VARIATION TIP: "Meatballs" without the pumpkin sauce can be served as appetizers, added to soups and stews, or simmered for 10 to 15 minutes with a jar of pasta sauce and used in sandwiches. Make an extra batch, and freeze until needed, or up to 3 months.

Per Serving: Calories: 788; Total fat: 28g; Saturated fat: 13g; Protein: 24g; Total carbs: 111g; Fiber: 14g; Sugar: 6g; Sodium: 976mg

Bacon and Chive Oatmeal

PREP TIME: 20 MINUTES • COOK TIME: 10 MINUTES

Oatmeal is a stick-to-your-ribs breakfast. Most people expect it to be sweet, but this savory version, topped with fresh chives and a smattering of bacon, will give you an entirely new appreciation of oatmeal. SERVES 4

3 cups whole milk

1 teaspoon sea salt

2 cups gluten-free old-fashioned oats

¾ cup chopped fresh chives

10 bacon slices, cooked, drained, and crumbled

1. In a large saucepan, combine the milk and salt. Bring to a boil over high heat.

2. Stir in the oats.

3. Reduce the heat to medium. Cook, stirring occasionally, for 5 minutes, or until the oatmeal has thickened. Remove from the heat. Let cool for 10 minutes.

4. In a small bowl, stir together the bacon and chives. Sprinkle evenly over the cooled oatmeal.

STORAGE: Put in an airtight container. Refrigerate for up to 5 days, or freeze for up to 3 months.

THAWING AND REHEATING: To reheat individual servings of frozen oatmeal, put in a microwave-safe bowl, and add 1 tablespoon milk. Microwave on high power for 1 minute. Stir and heat for 1 more minute. Stir before serving. To reheat refrigerated oatmeal, reduce the time to 30 seconds, stir, and heat for 30 more seconds, if needed.

VARIATION TIP: For Southwestern-style oatmeal, prepare the oatmeal as directed in steps 1 through 3. Top each serving with 2 tablespoons sautéed onion, ¼ cup whole kernel corn, and 1 tablespoon shredded Mexican-style cheese. Serve with avocado slices.

- -

Per Serving: Calories: 377; Total fat: 17g; Saturated fat: 7g; Protein: 20g; Total carbs: 35g; Fiber: 4g; Sugar: 9g; Sodium: 1,105mg

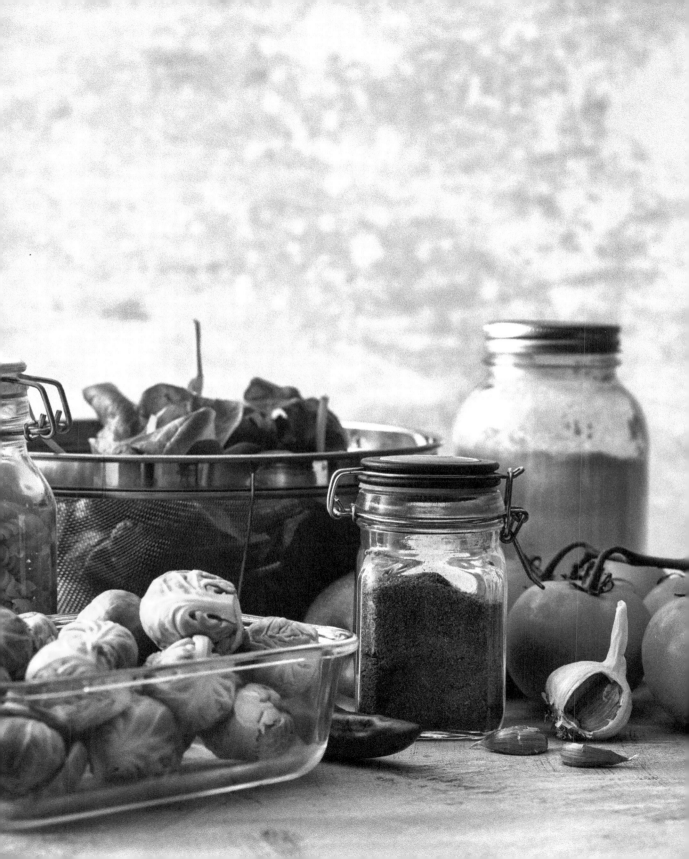

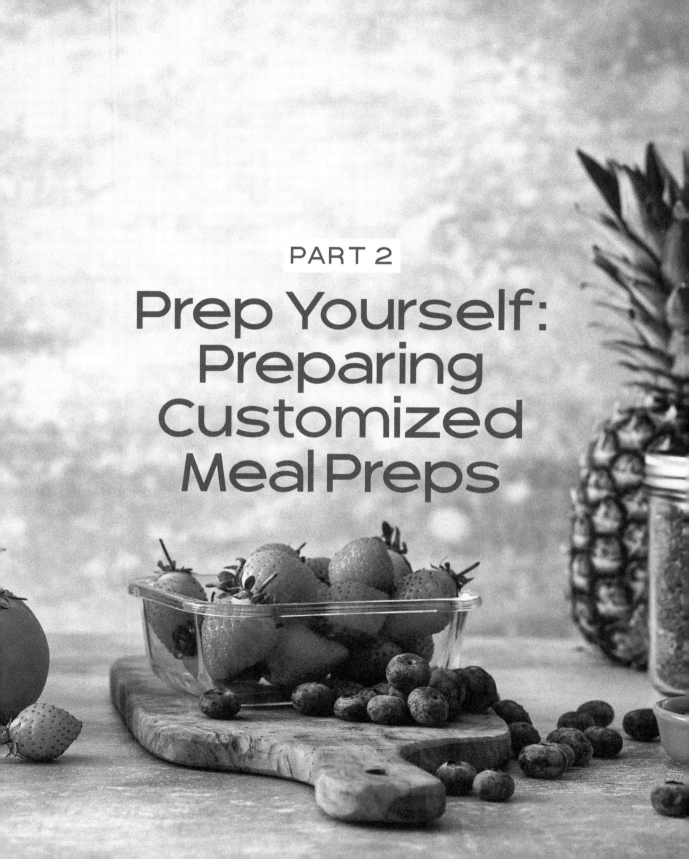

PART 2

Prep Yourself: Preparing Customized Meal Preps

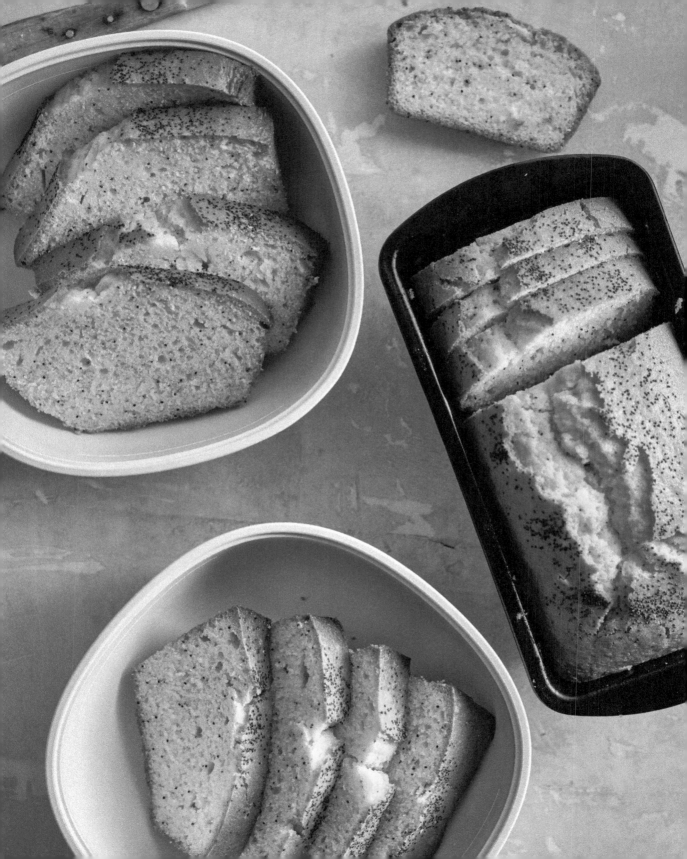

Rise and Shine:
Breaking for Breakfast

‹‹ Lemon–Poppy Seed Bread, page 158

Ham and Cheese Crêpes

PREP TIME: 20 MINUTES • COOK TIME: 20 TO 25 MINUTES

Crêpes are a specialty of Brittany, a northwestern region of France. Savory versions made with buckwheat, a crop ideally suited for growth in the area's rugged conditions, are known as galettes. These savory crêpes are inspired by galettes and overflow with ham, cheese, and sautéed vegetables. SERVES 4

2 large eggs, beaten

¾ cup whole milk

¼ cup water

4 tablespoons (½ stick) salted butter, melted, divided

1 cup all-purpose gluten-free one-to-one baking flour

½ teaspoon sea salt

1 yellow onion, chopped

1 (8-ounce) container sliced cremini mushrooms

Nonstick cooking spray, for coating the skillet

2 cups diced cooked ham

1 cup shredded mild Cheddar cheese

1. In a large bowl, whisk together the eggs, milk, water, and 2 tablespoons of butter until blended.

2. Add the flour and salt. Using a handheld mixer, mix on medium speed for about 3 minutes, or until well blended. Turn off the mixer.

3. In a medium skillet, combine the remaining 2 tablespoons of butter, the onion, and mushrooms. Cook, stirring frequently, over medium heat for 5 to 7 minutes, or until the onion is translucent. Remove from the heat. Transfer to a plate. Wipe out the skillet.

4. Spray the skillet with cooking spray, and heat over medium heat.

5. Making 1 crêpe at a time, add ¾ cup of the batter to the skillet. Cook, tilting the skillet to spread the batter evenly, for 2 to 3 minutes, or until lightly browned. Flip, and cook for 1 minute, or until lightly browned on the other side. Transfer to a work surface. Repeat 3 more times for 4 medium crêpes. Turn off the heat.

6. Add ½ cup of ham and ¼ cup of cheese to each crêpe.

7. Spoon ⅓ cup of the onion and mushroom mixture on top.

8. Starting at one end, roll each crêpe jelly roll–style.

STORAGE: Put in an airtight container. Refrigerate for up to 4 days, or freeze for up to 2 months.

THAWING AND REHEATING: Thaw in the refrigerator overnight. To reheat individual crêpes, put on a microwave-safe plate. Microwave on 50 percent power for 1 minute.

SUBSTITUTION TIP: Add 1 cup diced cooked turkey or chicken instead of ham. Try sautéed spinach and bacon for a twist.

Per Serving: Calories: 511; Total fat: 29g; Saturated fat: 16g; Protein: 31g; Total carbs: 32g; Fiber: 2g; Sugar: 6g; Sodium: 1,085mg

Eggs Florentine

PREP TIME: 15 MINUTES • COOK TIME: 35 TO 40 MINUTES

This quiche-like egg bake blends frozen spinach with two cheeses. Cottage cheese adds creaminess, while goat cheese lends a mellow bite. Top with leftover salsa for added flavor. SERVES 4

Nonstick cooking spray, for coating the baking dish

1 (10-ounce) package frozen chopped spinach, thawed and drained

8 large eggs, beaten

1 yellow onion, diced

1 (15-ounce) container low-fat cottage cheese

1 cup crumbled goat cheese

4 tablespoons (½ stick) unsalted butter, melted

1 teaspoon Italian seasoning

½ teaspoon sea salt

½ teaspoon freshly ground black pepper

1. Preheat the oven to 350°F. Coat a 9-by-13-inch baking dish with cooking spray.

2. Put the thawed spinach in a strainer, and press using a paper towel until all the water is removed. This helps prevent the eggs from becoming soggy.

3. In a large bowl, whisk together the eggs, onion, cottage cheese, goat cheese, and butter to blend.

4. Add the Italian seasoning, salt, and pepper. Whisk to combine.

5. Stir in the spinach.

6. Pour the egg mixture into the prepared baking dish.

7. Transfer the baking dish to the oven, and bake for 35 to 40 minutes, or until a knife inserted into the center of the egg mixture comes out clean. Remove from the oven. Let cool for 20 minutes.

STORAGE: Tightly wrap the baking dish in aluminum foil, or put the eggs in an airtight container. Refrigerate for up to 4 days, or freeze for up to 2 months.

THAWING AND REHEATING: Thaw in the refrigerator overnight. To reheat individual servings, wrap in a damp paper towel. Microwave on 50 percent power for 45 seconds. Heat for 15 to 30 more seconds, if needed.

Per Serving: Calories: 438; Total fat: 30g; Saturated fat: 16g; Protein: 32g; Total carbs: 11g; Fiber: 3g; Sugar: 6g; Sodium: 945mg

Three-Cheese Omelets with Bacon

PREP TIME: 15 MINUTES • COOK TIME: 20 TO 25 MINUTES

This fluffy omelet gets extra flavor from a blend of three cheeses. Adjust the heat level of the finished dish using hot or mild sausage, or switch up the cheese for your favorite blend. **SERVES 4**

8 bacon slices

9 large eggs, beaten

¼ cup whole milk

1 teaspoon sea salt

½ teaspoon freshly ground black pepper

¼ cup shredded sharp Cheddar cheese

¼ cup shredded Monterey Jack cheese

¼ cup shredded Parmesan cheese

8 tablespoons (1 stick) unsalted butter, divided

1. In a large skillet, cook the bacon over medium heat, turning every 3 minutes, for 7 to 10 minutes, or until crispy. Remove from the heat. Transfer to paper towels to drain and cool. Crumble the bacon.

2. In a large bowl, whisk together the eggs, milk, salt, and pepper until blended.

3. Add the Cheddar cheese, Monterey Jack cheese, and Parmesan cheese. Stir to combine.

4. In a medium skillet, melt 2 tablespoons of butter completely over medium heat.

5. Add one-fourth of the egg mixture. Cook, lifting the edges using a spatula to allow uncooked egg to flow underneath, for 2 to 3 minutes, or until the eggs are creamy and set.

6. Place one-fourth of the bacon down the center of the omelet. Using the spatula, fold the omelet in half. Slide the spatula underneath the omelet, and flip onto a plate. Repeat with the remaining butter, egg mixture, and bacon to make 4 omelets. Turn off the heat.

STORAGE: Tightly wrap each omelet in wax paper or parchment paper before putting in an airtight container. Refrigerate for up to 5 days, or freeze for up to 2 months.

CONTINUED ⟶

THAWING AND REHEATING: Thaw in the refrigerator overnight. To reheat, wrap an omelet in a paper towel, and put on a microwave-safe plate. Microwave on high power for 45 seconds, flip, and heat for 15 more seconds, if needed.

PREPARATION TIP: Crumbled cooked bacon can be frozen in an airtight container for up to 3 months. Cook an extra package to save time during future recipe preps.

Per Serving: Calories: 544; Total fat: 48g; Saturated fat: 24g; Protein: 26g; Total carbs: 3g; Fiber: 0g; Sugar: 1g; Sodium: 1,207mg

Frozen Fruit Cups

PREP TIME: 15 MINUTES

Frozen fruit cups are a cool, refreshing change of pace for breakfast, snacks, or dessert. Substitute your favorite fruits and fruit juices, or use leftover fruit to create new flavor combinations. **SERVES 4**

1½ cups seedless red grapes

1 (15-ounce) can peach slices in juice, drained and diced

1 (15-ounce) can pineapple chunks in juice, strained, 1 cup juice reserved

2 large bananas, sliced

¼ cup sugar

6 ounces canned frozen orange juice concentrate, thawed

¼ cup freshly squeezed lemon juice

1. In a large bowl, stir together the grapes, peaches, pineapple chunks, bananas, sugar, reserved pineapple juice, orange juice concentrate, and lemon juice until well mixed.

2. Evenly divide the fruit and juice among 4 (8-ounce) Mason jars. Seal the jars.

STORAGE: Freeze for up to 3 months.

THAWING AND REHEATING: Thaw for 1 to 2 hours at room temperature, or refrigerate overnight to thaw before serving.

VARIATION TIP: Add 1 cup chopped maraschino cherries, 1 cup halved seedless green grapes, or 1 cup fresh blueberries to the mix.

Per Serving: Calories: 278; Total fat: 1g; Saturated fat: 0g; Protein: 3g; Total carbs: 72g; Fiber: 5g; Sugar: 59g; Sodium: 8mg

Lemon-Poppy Seed Bread

PREP TIME: 20 MINUTES • COOK TIME: 40 MINUTES

Start the day on a sweet note with this quick bread. There's no involved prep, no waiting for the loaves to rise, and no long baking time—only lemony goodness. MAKES 2 LOAVES

Nonstick cooking spray, for coating the loaf pans

3 cups all-purpose gluten-free one-to-one baking flour

1½ teaspoons baking powder

½ teaspoon sea salt

2¼ cups sugar

3 large eggs, beaten

1⅛ cups canola oil

1½ teaspoons vanilla extract

1½ teaspoons lemon extract

1½ cups whole milk

1½ teaspoons poppy seeds

1. Preheat the oven to 350°F. Coat 2 (9-by-5-inch) loaf pans with cooking spray.

2. In a large bowl, whisk together the flour, baking powder, and salt to combine.

3. In another large bowl, combine the sugar, eggs, and oil. Using a handheld mixer, beat on medium speed for about 3 minutes, or until the sugar is light and fluffy.

4. Blend in the vanilla and lemon extract.

5. Alternating between each addition and mixing thoroughly after each, add the flour mixture and milk.

6. Turn off the mixer. Stir in the poppy seeds.

7. Fill each prepared loaf pan halfway with the batter.

8. Transfer the loaf pans to the oven, and bake for 35 to 40 minutes, or until a knife inserted into the center of a loaf comes out clean. Remove from the oven.

STORAGE: Put the loaves in airtight containers. Store at room temperature for 2 days, refrigerate for up to 1 week, or freeze for up to 3 months.

THAWING AND REHEATING: Thaw the bread at room temperature for several hours or overnight in the refrigerator. To reheat individual slices, loosely wrap in a paper towel. Microwave on high power for 10 to 15 seconds.

Per Serving (1 slice or 1/8 loaf): Calories: 360; Total fat: 17g; Saturated fat: 2g; Protein: 4g; Total carbs: 47g; Fiber: 1g; Sugar: 29g; Sodium: 131mg

Carrot and Granola Muffins

PREP TIME: 20 MINUTES • COOK TIME: 20 MINUTES

Carrots and brown sugar give these moist muffins their sweetness, and the granola adds crunch. Use different granola blends to give these muffins a different taste each time you make them. **MAKES 12 MUFFINS**

Nonstick cooking spray, for coating the muffin tin

1½ cups gluten-free granola

1 cup packed light brown sugar

1 cup low-fat buttermilk

1¼ cups all-purpose gluten-free one-to-one baking flour

2 teaspoons baking powder

½ teaspoon baking soda

½ teaspoon ground allspice

2 large eggs, beaten

2 tablespoons canola oil

1 cup grated carrots

1. Preheat the oven to 400°F. Coat a 12-cup muffin tin with cooking spray.

2. In a large bowl, stir together the granola, sugar, and buttermilk. Let stand for 5 minutes.

3. In another large bowl, whisk together the flour, baking powder, baking soda, and allspice until blended.

4. Stir the eggs, oil, and carrots into the granola mixture.

5. To make the batter, add the flour mixture, and stir just until blended.

6. Spoon the batter into the prepared muffin cups, filling each two-thirds full.

7. Transfer the muffin tin to the oven, and bake for 20 minutes, or until a knife inserted into the center of a muffin comes out clean. Remove from the oven.

STORAGE: Put in an airtight container. Store at room temperature for up to 3 days, refrigerate for up to 1 week, or freeze for up to 3 months. If freezing, wrap each muffin individually in aluminum foil before putting in an airtight freezer-safe container.

THAWING AND REHEATING: Let the frozen muffins sit at room temperature for 1 hour, or wrap in a paper towel and microwave on high power for 1 minute.

INGREDIENT TIP: Always read granola labels carefully because many are not gluten-free.

Per Serving (1 muffin): Calories: 216; Total fat: 5g; Saturated fat: 1g; Protein: 4g; Total carbs: 38g; Fiber: 2g; Sugar: 21g; Sodium: 173mg

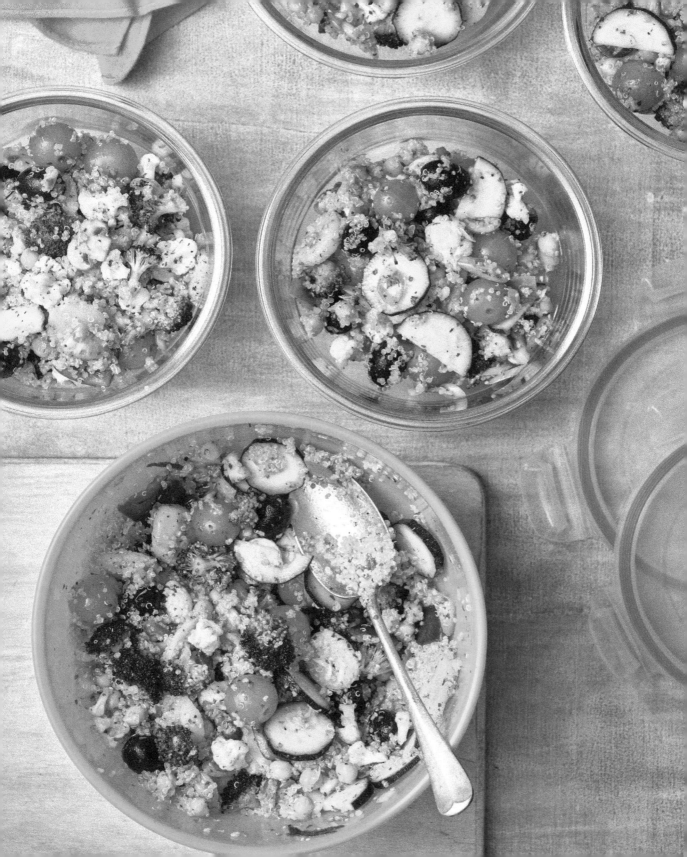

Take Time to Nourish: Lunch and Dinner

‹‹ Marinated Garden Vegetable Bowl with Quinoa, page 170

Curried Tuna Salad

PREP TIME: 15 MINUTES • COOK TIME: 25 MINUTES

Tuna salad is an American dish created in the 19th century to conserve food. Cooks often mixed leftover meat, mayonnaise, and other ingredients for a quick meal. My version features a dash of heat from the curry and yellow rice. **SERVES 4**

For the rice
2 cups chicken broth
1 cup long-grain white rice
½ cup chopped yellow onion
1 tablespoon minced garlic
½ cup chopped bell pepper, any color
½ teaspoon ground turmeric
½ teaspoon freshly ground black pepper
½ teaspoon sea salt

For the tuna salad
3 (6½-ounce) cans chunk tuna, drained
½ cup full-fat mayonnaise
2 tablespoons freshly squeezed lemon juice
1 to 2 teaspoons curry powder
½ cup chopped celery
½ cup diced yellow onion
½ cup chopped fresh parsley
½ cup sliced black olives

To make the rice

1. In a large saucepan, combine the broth, rice, onion, garlic, bell pepper, turmeric, pepper, and salt. Bring to a boil over high heat.

2. Reduce the heat to low. Cover the pan, and simmer for 15 minutes, or until the rice is fluffy, tender, and golden yellow. Remove from the heat. Let cool.

To make the tuna salad

3. In a large bowl, stir together the tuna, mayonnaise, lemon juice, curry powder, celery, onion, parsley, and olives until well mixed.

4. Add 3 cups of the cooled rice, and stir to combine.

STORAGE: Put in an airtight container. Refrigerate for up to 4 days. Freezing salads containing mayonnaise is not recommended since ingredients will separate.

SUBSTITUTION TIP: Crab, imitation crab (read the label to be sure it's gluten-free), chopped cooked shrimp, or diced cooked chicken can be used instead of tuna. Create a new flavor profile for this salad by adding any of the following: sliced water chestnuts, diced green bell pepper, or chopped dill pickle.

Per Serving: Calories: 513; Total fat: 24g; Saturated fat: 4g; Protein: 27g; Total carbs: 47g; Fiber: 3g; Sugar: 4g; Sodium: 1,158mg

Spicy Salsa Chili

PREP TIME: 20 MINUTES • COOK TIME: 30 TO 35 MINUTES

Choose mild, medium, or spicy salsa to change the heat level of this dish. Shredded cheese, sour cream, chopped jalapeños, and even black olives make for excellent toppings. **SERVES 4**

2 tablespoons extra-virgin olive oil

1½ pounds 80/20 ground beef

1 yellow onion, chopped

2 tablespoons minced garlic

2 (1-pound) jars salsa

1 (15-ounce) can kidney beans, drained and rinsed

¼ cup low-fat sour cream (optional)

¼ cup shredded Mexican-style cheese (optional)

1. In a large saucepan, heat the oil over medium heat.

2. Add the beef, onion, and garlic. Cook, stirring to break up the beef, for 5 to 7 minutes, or until the onion is translucent and the beef is beginning to brown. Drain the beef mixture and return to the pan.

3. Stir in the salsa and beans.

4. Increase the heat to high. Bring to a boil, stirring constantly.

5. Reduce the heat to low. Simmer, stirring occasionally, for 20 minutes, or until the beef has cooked through and the chili is hot. Remove from the heat.

6. Serve the chili with the sour cream (if using) and cheese (if using).

STORAGE: Put in airtight containers. Refrigerate for up to 4 days, or freeze for up to 3 months. Refrigerate the sour cream and shredded cheese (if using) separately in airtight containers for up to 5 days.

THAWING AND REHEATING: Thaw in the refrigerator overnight. To reheat individual servings, put the chili in a microwave-safe bowl, and cover with a paper towel. Microwave on 50 percent power for 1 minute. Stir and heat for 30 more seconds, if needed.

VARIATION TIP: For an even spicier chili, add 1 teaspoon chili powder and ½ teaspoon red pepper flakes while browning the beef.

- -

Per Serving: Calories: 689; Total fat: 42g; Saturated fat: 14g; Protein: 41g; Total carbs: 39g; Fiber: 10g; Sugar: 14g; Sodium: 921mg

Sausage, Spinach, and Chickpea Soup

PREP TIME: 15 MINUTES • COOK TIME: 40 TO 45 MINUTES

According to a theory by archaeologist John Speth, the origins of soup might have been in the Neanderthal era. This modern version comes together quickly but tastes like it has simmered for hours. SERVES 4

1 pound Italian sausage links, casings removed

1 teaspoon extra-virgin olive oil

1 yellow onion, diced

2 tablespoons minced garlic

1 tablespoon Italian seasoning

1 teaspoon sea salt

½ teaspoon freshly ground black pepper

½ teaspoon red pepper flakes

1 (10-ounce) package chopped frozen spinach

1 (15-ounce) can chickpeas, drained and rinsed

1½ cups beef broth

1 (28-ounce) can Italian-style diced tomatoes

1 tablespoon cornstarch

1 tablespoon water

½ cup shredded Parmesan cheese

1. In a large skillet, cook the sausage over medium heat, stirring often to crumble the meat, for 7 to 8 minutes, or until no longer pink. Remove from the heat. Drain.

2. In a large saucepan, combine the oil, onion, and garlic. Cook over medium heat for 5 to 7 minutes, or until the onion is soft and translucent.

3. Add the cooked sausage, Italian seasoning, salt, black pepper, red pepper flakes, spinach, chickpeas, broth, and tomatoes with their juices. Stir to combine, and bring to a boil.

4. Reduce the heat to low. Cover the pan, and simmer, stirring occasionally, for 20 minutes, or until the soup begins to thicken.

5. To make a slurry, in a small bowl, whisk together the cornstarch and water until blended.

6. Stir the slurry into the soup. Simmer for 5 more minutes, or until the soup has thickened. Remove from the heat.

7. Sprinkle the cheese on top to serve.

STORAGE: Put in airtight containers. Refrigerate for up to 5 days, or freeze for up to 3 months.

THAWING AND REHEATING: Thaw in the refrigerator overnight. To reheat individual servings, put the soup in a microwave-safe bowl, and cover with a paper towel. Microwave on high power for 30 seconds. Stir and heat for 30 to 45 more seconds, if needed.

SUBSTITUTION TIP: Substitute 2½ cups torn and washed fresh spinach for the frozen spinach. Add it with the sausage and seasonings.

- -

Per Serving: Calories: 436; Total fat: 17g; Saturated fat: 6g; Protein: 33g; Total carbs: 41g; Fiber: 12g; Sugar: 10g; Sodium: 1,721mg

Spicy Chicken with Peanut Sauce

PREP TIME: 30 MINUTES • COOK TIME: 40 TO 45 MINUTES

The smooth creaminess of peanut butter combines with red pepper flakes for a hint of heat. A touch of ginger gives this mouthwatering dish a deeper flavor. **SERVES 4**

1 cup dried lentils, rinsed

3 cups water

1 tablespoon gluten-free soy sauce or tamari

2 tablespoons sugar

2 tablespoons distilled white vinegar

¼ cup creamy peanut butter

3 tablespoons sesame oil, divided

2 tablespoons canola oil

3 scallions, white parts only, chopped

1 tablespoon minced garlic

1 tablespoon minced peeled fresh ginger

1 teaspoon red pepper flakes

1 pound boneless, skinless chicken breasts, diced

1. In a large saucepan, combine the lentils and water. Bring to a boil over high heat.

2. Reduce the heat to low. Cover the pan, and simmer, stirring occasionally, for 18 to 20 minutes, or until the lentils are tender. Remove from the heat. Let sit for 5 minutes before using. Drain any excess water.

3. Meanwhile, to make the peanut sauce, in a food processor or blender, combine the soy sauce, sugar, vinegar, and peanut butter. Process for 5 to 10 seconds, or until blended.

4. In a medium skillet, combine 1 tablespoon of sesame oil, the canola oil, scallions, garlic, ginger, and red pepper flakes. Cook over medium heat for 2 to 3 minutes, or until the scallions are translucent and tender.

5. Stir in the chicken and remaining 2 tablespoons of sesame oil. Cook, stirring constantly, for 5 to 7 minutes, or until the chicken is cooked through and no longer pink. Remove from the heat.

6. Stir in the peanut sauce and lentils to combine.

STORAGE: Put in airtight containers. Refrigerate for up to 4 days, or freeze for up to 3 months.

THAWING AND REHEATING: Thaw in the refrigerator overnight. To heat individual servings, put in a microwave-safe dish, and loosely cover with a paper towel. Microwave on high power for 45 seconds. Stir and heat for 15 to 30 more seconds, if needed.

SUBSTITUTION TIP: Replace the chicken with an equal amount of chopped cooked pork or shrimp. One pound of snow peas or sugar snap peas can be added to the peanut mixture.

- -

Per Serving: Calories: 577; Total fat: 28g; Saturated fat: 4g; Protein: 41g; Total carbs: 42g; Fiber: 6g; Sugar: 9g; Sodium: 286mg

Cheese-Stuffed Shells

PREP TIME: 20 MINUTES • COOK TIME: 50 MINUTES

Three cheeses—cottage, Parmesan, and mozzarella—are blended, packed in shells, and topped with a simple sauce loaded with flavorful herbs. Elegant enough to serve to guests, this meal will appeal to all ages and all of your senses. SERVES 4

For the shells

16 gluten-free jumbo pasta shells

For the sauce

2 tablespoons extra-virgin olive oil

1 yellow onion, diced

2 tablespoons minced garlic

1 (28-ounce) can diced tomatoes

1 (8-ounce) can tomato sauce

1 teaspoon dried oregano

1 teaspoon dried basil

1 teaspoon dried rosemary

1 teaspoon sea salt

1 teaspoon light brown sugar

For the stuffing

1 (15-ounce) container full-fat cottage cheese

1 cup shredded mozzarella cheese

½ cup shredded Parmesan cheese

1 large egg, beaten

2 teaspoons Italian seasoning

1 teaspoon garlic powder

1 teaspoon sea salt

To make the shells

1. Cook the shells for 4 minutes less than the package directions indicate. Drain.

To make the sauce

2. In a large skillet, combine the oil, onion, and garlic. Cook over medium heat, stirring often, for 5 to 7 minutes, or until the onion is tender and translucent.

3. Stir in the tomatoes with their juices, tomato sauce, oregano, basil, rosemary, salt, and sugar until combined. Bring to a boil, stirring occasionally.

4. Reduce the heat to low. Simmer for 10 minutes, or until the sauce has slightly thickened. Remove from the heat.

To make the stuffing

5. In medium bowl, stir together the cottage cheese, mozzarella cheese, Parmesan cheese, and egg until thoroughly mixed.

6. Stir in the Italian seasoning, garlic powder, salt, and pepper to blend.

7. Preheat the oven to 375°F. Coat a 9-by-13-inch baking dish with cooking spray.

8. Spoon 2 to 3 tablespoons of the stuffing into each shell.

9. Arrange the stuffed shells in the prepared baking dish.

1 teaspoon freshly ground black pepper

Nonstick cooking spray, for coating the baking dish

10. Evenly spread the sauce over the stuffed shells. Cover the dish with aluminum foil.

11. Transfer the baking dish to the oven, and bake for 30 minutes, or until the filling is warmed through and the shells are soft.

STORAGE: Refrigerate the shells, covered with sauce, in an airtight container for up to 5 days, or freeze for up to 3 months.

THAWING AND REHEATING: Thaw in the refrigerator overnight. To reheat individual servings, put 4 shells in a microwave-safe dish, and loosely cover with a paper towel. Microwave on high power for 1 minute. Stir and heat for 30 more seconds, if needed.

VARIATION TIP: For an unstuffed version, cook rigatoni or penne according to the package directions. Stir together the filling and sauce to combine. Add the pasta and stir to coat. For a meaty version, add 1 pound cooked Italian sausage.

- -

Per Serving: Calories: 598; Total fat: 24g; Saturated fat: 9g; Protein: 30g; Total carbs: 67g; Fiber: 7g; Sugar: 14g; Sodium: 1,723mg

Marinated Garden Vegetable Bowl with Quinoa

PREP TIME: 10 MINUTES • COOK TIME: 20 MINUTES

Crunchy summer vegetables and fluffy quinoa star in this delightful salad. The trick to removing the bitter taste from quinoa is to rinse it thoroughly to remove its natural saponin coating before cooking.

SERVES 4

1 cup quinoa, rinsed

1¾ cups water

½ cup chopped green
   bell pepper

1 cup cherry tomatoes

1 cup sliced mushrooms

¾ cup sliced water
   chestnuts, drained

1 zucchini, thinly sliced

1 cup sliced black olives

1 cup chopped cauliflower

1 cup chopped
   broccoli florets

6 scallions, white parts only,
   thinly sliced

1 cup chickpeas, drained
   and rinsed

2 cups Italian Dressing
   (page 182)

1. In a large saucepan, combine the quinoa and water. Bring to a boil over high heat.

2. Reduce the heat to low. Cover the pan, and simmer for 18 to 20 minutes, or until the quinoa is soft. Remove from the heat. Let rest for 5 minutes.

3. In a large bowl, stir together the bell pepper, tomatoes, mushrooms, water chestnuts, zucchini, olives, cauliflower, broccoli, scallions, and chickpeas.

4. Add the Italian dressing, and stir until the mixture is thoroughly coated.

5. Stir in the quinoa. Refrigerate to let the vegetables marinate in the dressing and the salad chill. Serve cold.

STORAGE: Put in an airtight container. Refrigerate for up to 5 days. Freezing is not recommended, since the vegetables will become mushy.

SUBSTITUTION TIP: Any of the following vegetables can be added: 1 cup diced celery; 1 (15-ounce) can kidney beans, drained and rinsed; 1 pound fresh snow peas; 1 cup thinly sliced carrot.

Per Serving: Calories: 466; Total fat: 18g; Saturated fat: 2g; Protein: 14g; Total carbs: 64g; Fiber: 13g; Sugar: 8g; Sodium: 280mg

Chicken Cacciatore

Hearty chunks of steamy seasoned chicken and tomatoes make this recipe perfect for a chilly day. The quinoa adds a nutty flavor and provides an updated touch to an old favorite. SERVES 4

1 cup quinoa, rinsed

1¾ cups water

¼ cup extra-virgin olive oil

1 pound boneless, skinless chicken breasts, cut into chunks

½ cup diced green bell pepper

½ cup diced yellow onion

1 tablespoon minced garlic

1 (14½-ounce) can tomato sauce

1 (5-ounce) can tomato paste

1 tablespoon Italian seasoning

½ teaspoon sea salt

½ teaspoon freshly ground black pepper

1 (8-ounce) package cremini mushrooms, sliced

½ cup shredded Italian cheese blend (optional)

1. In a large saucepan, combine the quinoa and water. Bring to a boil over high heat.

2. Reduce the heat to low. Cover the pan, and simmer for 18 to 20 minutes, or until the quinoa is soft. Remove from the heat. Let rest for 5 minutes.

3. Meanwhile, in a large skillet, combine the oil, chicken, bell pepper, onion, and garlic. Cook over medium heat, stirring for 5 to 7 minutes, or until the onion is tender and translucent.

4. In a small bowl, stir together the tomato sauce, tomato paste, Italian seasoning, salt, and pepper until blended. Stir into the chicken mixture.

5. Add the mushrooms, and stir to combine.

6. Reduce the heat to low. Cover the skillet, and simmer, stirring occasionally, for 20 minutes, or until the chicken and mushrooms are tender. Remove from the heat.

7. Stir in the quinoa, and top with the cheese (if using) to serve.

STORAGE: Put in airtight containers. Refrigerate for up to 4 days, or freeze up to 3 months.

THAWING AND REHEATING: Thaw in the refrigerator overnight. To reheat individual servings, put in a microwave-safe dish, and cover with a paper towel. Microwave on high power for 1 minute. Stir and heat for 30 seconds to 1 minute more, if needed.

Per Serving: Calories: 472; Total fat: 19g; Saturated fat: 3g; Protein: 36g; Total carbs: 43g; Fiber: 8g; Sugar: 9g; Sodium: 495mg

Tomato Soup

PREP TIME: 15 MINUTES • COOK TIME: 35 MINUTES

No one has to know the secret: this thick, creamy, easy soup is ready in less than an hour. It will become a fast favorite for lunch or dinner. Feel free to sprinkle the soup with some shredded mild Cheddar cheese before serving. **SERVES 4**

2 tablespoons extra-virgin olive oil

2 tablespoons minced garlic

1 yellow onion, diced

2 celery stalks, diced

1 (28-ounce) can Italian-style diced tomatoes

1 (5-ounce) can tomato paste

1 tablespoon Italian seasoning

1 teaspoon sugar

2 cups whole milk

2 tablespoons all-purpose gluten-free one-to-one baking flour

1. In a large saucepan, combine the oil, garlic, onion, and celery. Cook over medium heat for 5 to 7 minutes, or until the onion is tender and translucent.

2. Stir in the tomatoes with their juices, tomato paste, Italian seasoning, and sugar. Bring to a boil.

3. Reduce the heat to low. Simmer, stirring occasionally, for 10 minutes.

4. In medium bowl, whisk together the milk and flour until blended. Stir into the soup. Simmer, stirring often, for 10 more minutes, or until slightly thickened and warmed through. Remove from the heat.

STORAGE: Put in an airtight container. Refrigerate for up to 5 days, or freeze for up to 3 months.

THAWING AND REHEATING: Thaw in the refrigerator overnight. To reheat individual servings, put the soup in a microwave-safe bowl, and loosely cover with a paper towel. Microwave on high power for 45 seconds. Stir and heat for 30 more seconds, if needed.

PREPARATION TIP: Using an immersion blender, blend the soup after cooking for a thicker, creamier texture.

Per Serving: Calories: 230; Total fat: 11g; Saturated fat: 3g; Protein: 8g; Total carbs: 28g; Fiber: 2g; Sugar: 13g; Sodium: 878mg

Chili Pie
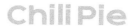

PREP TIME: 15 MINUTES • COOK TIME: 1 HOUR 5 MINUTES

The cheesy rice crust of this pie provides the perfect backdrop for the seasoned bean and vegetable filling. If you have extra salsa, add ½ cup to the bean mixture before baking. SERVES 4

For the crust

Nonstick cooking spray, for coating the baking dish

3½ cups water

1½ cups long-grain white rice

¼ cup shredded mild Cheddar cheese

1 large egg, beaten

½ teaspoon sea salt

For the filling

2 tablespoons extra-virgin olive oil

½ cup diced yellow onion

½ cup diced green bell pepper

2 tablespoons minced garlic

1 (15-ounce) can chili beans, drained

1 (14½-ounce) can diced tomatoes, drained

1 teaspoon cayenne pepper

1 teaspoon chili powder

1 tablespoon cornstarch

1 teaspoon water

½ cup shredded sharp Cheddar cheese

To make the crust

1. Preheat the oven to 350°F. Coat a 9-by-9-inch baking dish with cooking spray.

2. In a large saucepan, combine the water and rice. Bring to a boil over medium heat. Stir, and cover the pan.

3. Reduce the heat to low. Simmer, stirring occasionally, for 20 minutes, or until the rice is tender. Remove from the heat. Let cool for 10 minutes.

4. In a large bowl, stir together the rice, cheese, egg, and salt.

5. Press the rice mixture into the bottom and up the sides of the prepared baking dish.

6. Transfer the baking dish to the oven, and bake for 10 minutes. Remove from the oven, leaving the oven on.

To make the filling

7. In a large skillet, combine the oil, onion, bell pepper, and garlic. Cook over medium heat for 5 to 7 minutes, or until the onion is tender and translucent. Remove from the heat. Transfer to a large bowl.

8. To the onion mixture, add the chili beans, tomatoes, cayenne, and chili powder.

9. To make a slurry, in a small bowl, stir together the cornstarch and water until the cornstarch dissolves.

CONTINUED ····→

10. Blend the slurry into the onion-bean mixture.

11. Pour the filling over the prepared crust.

12. Return the baking dish to the oven, and bake for 20 to 25 minutes, or until the filling is hot and bubbly.

13. Sprinkle with the cheese. Bake for 5 more minutes, or until the cheese melts. Remove from the oven.

STORAGE: Tightly wrap the pie in aluminum foil, or put in an airtight container. Refrigerate for up to 5 days, or freeze for up to 3 months.

THAWING AND REHEATING: Thaw in the refrigerator overnight. To heat individual servings, put on a microwave-safe dish. Microwave on high power for 45 seconds. Heat for 30 more seconds, if needed.

VARIATION TIP: Delicious toppings for this pie include additional shredded cheese, sliced black olives, and sour cream.

Per Serving: Calories: 571; Total fat: 17g; Saturated fat: 6g; Protein: 20g; Total carbs: 85g; Fiber: 4g; Sugar: 4g; Sodium: 784mg

Unstuffed Bell Peppers

PREP TIME: 15 MINUTES • COOK TIME: ABOUT 1 HOUR

Love traditional stuffed peppers but don't have the time for all the work? This unstuffed version hits the spot. SERVES 4

3½ cups water

1½ cups basmati rice

Nonstick cooking spray, for coating the baking dish

2 tablespoons salted butter

2 green bell peppers, diced

1 white onion, chopped

1 (28-ounce) can Italian-style diced tomatoes

1 cup shredded mild Cheddar cheese

2 teaspoons Italian seasoning

1 teaspoon sea salt

1 teaspoon freshly ground black pepper

½ cup gluten-free bread crumbs

1. In a large saucepan, combine the water and rice. Bring to a boil over medium heat. Stir, and cover the pan.

2. Reduce the heat to low. Simmer, stirring occasionally, for 20 minutes, or until the rice is tender. Remove from the heat. Let cool.

3. Preheat the oven to 350°F. Coat a 9-by-9-inch baking dish with cooking spray.

4. In a medium skillet, melt the butter over medium heat.

5. Add the bell peppers and onion. Cook, stirring, until the onion is translucent. Remove from the heat. Transfer to a large bowl.

6. To the bell pepper and onion mixture, add the rice, tomatoes, cheese, Italian seasoning, salt, and pepper. Stir until well blended.

7. Pour the rice mixture into the prepared baking dish.

8. Evenly sprinkle the bread crumbs on top.

9. Transfer the baking dish to the oven, and bake for 25 to 30 minutes, or until the peppers are tender. Remove from the oven.

STORAGE: Put in an airtight container. Refrigerate for up to 5 days, or freeze for up to 3 months.

THAWING AND REHEATING: Thaw in the refrigerator overnight. To reheat, put in a microwave-safe dish, and loosely cover with a paper towel. Microwave on low for 1 minute. Stir and heat for 30 more seconds, if needed.

Per Serving: Calories: 538; Total fat: 17g; Saturated fat: 10g; Protein: 16g; Total carbs: 81g; Fiber: 7g; Sugar: 9g; Sodium: 832mg

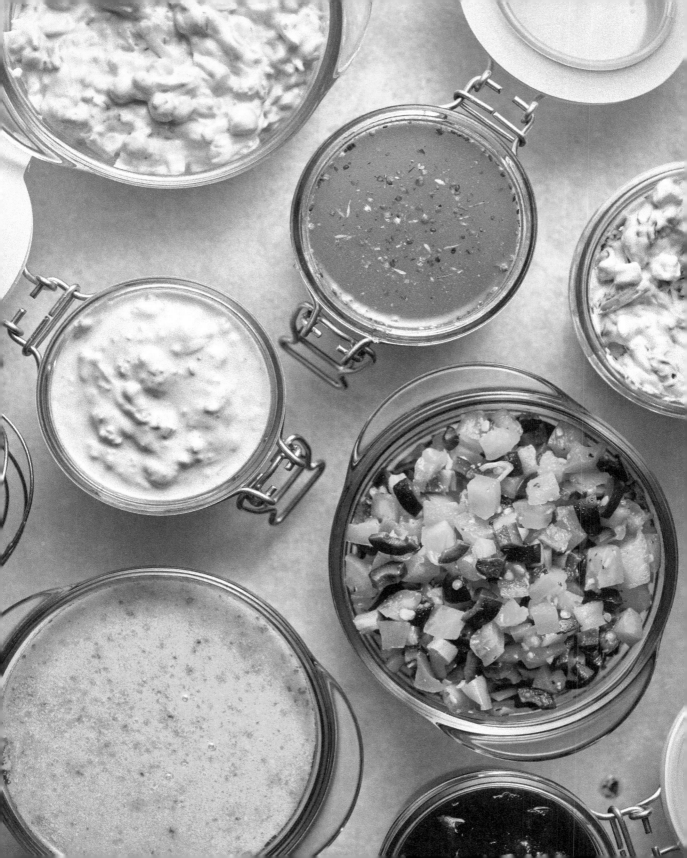

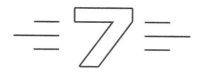

Recipes to Relish: Sauces, Dressings, and Dips

‹‹ Clockwise from top left: Scallion-Corn Dip, page 180; Italian Dressing, page 182; Spinach Dip, page 179; Black Olive Salsa, page 178; Blueberry Chutney, page 184; Creamy Balsamic Dressing, page 60; Creamy Blue Cheese Dressing, page 181

Black Olive Salsa

PREP TIME: 15 MINUTES, PLUS 4 HOURS TO CHILL

The origin of salsa dates back to the Aztecs and Incas, and the original version includes tomatoes and chilies. This recipe gets a different flavor from its olive base. It's the perfect dip with Spicy Tortilla Chips (page 189), or it makes for a tasty garnish for Cheese and Jalapeño Bake (page 56), Sheet Pan Steak Fajitas (page 57), or Eggs Florentine (page 154). **MAKES 2 CUPS**

3 large tomatoes, diced

1 (4½-ounce) can diced green chilies

1 (15-ounce) can pitted black olives, drained and diced

2 tablespoons canola oil

1 tablespoon distilled white vinegar

1 teaspoon minced garlic

½ teaspoon sea salt

½ teaspoon freshly ground black pepper

Gluten-free chips or crackers of choice, for serving

In a medium bowl, stir together the tomatoes, green chilies, olives, oil, vinegar, garlic, salt, and pepper until blended. Refrigerate for 4 hours to allow the flavors to meld before serving.

STORAGE: Put in an airtight container. Refrigerate for up to 5 days, or freeze for up to 3 months.

THAWING AND REHEATING: Thaw in the refrigerator for 2 to 3 hours before serving.

VARIATION TIP: For corn salsa, substitute 1 (15-ounce) can Southwestern-style whole kernel corn for the olives.

INGREDIENT TIP: Chose firm red tomatoes with no soft spots. Keep in mind tomatoes will continue to ripen after purchase. Keep tomatoes at room temperature, in a single layer, on the countertop and away from sunlight. Refrigerating causes a change in texture.

- -

Per Serving (¼ cup): Calories: 114; Total fat: 11g; Saturated fat: 2g; Protein: 1g; Total carbs: 5g; Fiber: 3g; Sugar: 2g; Sodium: 903mg

NUT-FREE

Spinach Dip

Serve this dish cold as a dip with chips or warmed as an appetizer with fresh chopped vegetables. The dip can be prepared with low-fat ingredients, if desired. For a fun presentation, sprinkle with shredded Cheddar cheese immediately before serving. **MAKES 2½ CUPS**

1 (10-ounce) package
   frozen spinach
½ cup full-fat cream cheese,
   at room temperature
½ cup full-fat sour cream
½ cup full-fat mayonnaise
½ cup diced yellow onion
1 teaspoon gluten-free
   Worcestershire sauce
1 teaspoon seasoned salt
Cut vegetables or
   gluten-free chips of choice,
   for dipping

1. Put the spinach in a microwave-safe bowl. Microwave on high power for 1 to 2 minutes, or until the spinach is mushy. Transfer to a strainer, and press on it using a paper towel until all the water is removed. Transfer to a large bowl.

2. Add the cream cheese, sour cream, mayonnaise, onion, Worcestershire sauce, and seasoned salt. Using a handheld mixer, beat on low speed for 3 to 4 minutes, or until blended. Turn off the mixer.

3. Serve the dip with vegetables or chips.

STORAGE: Put in an airtight container. Refrigerate for up to 5 days. Freezing is not recommended, because the texture and consistency will change if frozen.

PREPARATION TIP: Bake it. Preheat the oven to 325°F. Coat a 9-by-9-inch baking dish with cooking spray. Make the dip as directed, transfer to the prepared baking dish, and bake for 15 to 20 minutes, or until heated through.

VARIATION TIP: For a Southern-style spinach dip, add 1 (8-ounce) can sliced water chestnuts, drained, and top with 2 crumbled, cooked bacon slices.

Per Serving (2 tablespoons): Calories: 74; Total fat: 7g; Saturated fat: 2g; Protein: 1g; Total carbs: 2g; Fiber: 1g; Sugar: 1g; Sodium: 189mg

Scallion-Corn Dip

PREP TIME: 10 MINUTES, PLUS 2 HOURS TO CHILL

This dip can be served hot or cold. MAKES 3 CUPS

1 cup full-fat sour cream

1 cup full-fat mayonnaise

½ cup minced scallion, white and green parts divided

½ teaspoon sea salt

½ cup shredded sharp Cheddar cheese

1 (15¼-ounce) Southwestern-style whole-kernel corn, drained

Cut vegetables or gluten-free crackers of choice, for dipping

1. In a medium bowl, stir together the sour cream, mayonnaise, white parts of the scallion, and salt until blended.

2. Stir in the cheese and corn. Refrigerate for 2 hours to let the flavors meld.

3. Serve the dip with vegetables or crackers. Garnish with the green parts of the scallion, if desired.

STORAGE: Put in an airtight container. Refrigerate for up to 1 week. Freezing is not recommended, because the texture and consistency will change if frozen.

PREPARATION TIP: Bake it. Preheat the oven to 325°F. Coat a 9-by-9-inch baking dish with cooking spray. Make the dip as directed, and transfer to the prepared baking dish. Bake for 15 to 20 minutes, or until warmed and the cheese has melted.

- -

Per Serving (2 tablespoons): Calories: 102; Total fat: 10g; Saturated fat: 3g; Protein: 1g; Total carbs: 3g; Fiber: 0g; Sugar: 1g; Sodium: 155mg

Creamy Blue Cheese Dressing

PREP TIME: 10 MINUTES, PLUS 2 HOURS TO CHILL

Blue cheese is a sharp cheese with a salty bite. Because it is pungent, only a small amount is needed to add flavor to dishes. Feta can be substituted for blue cheese in this recipe. **MAKES 2 CUPS**

1 (1-pound) container full-fat plain yogurt

1 (4-ounce) package crumbled blue cheese

3 scallions, white parts only, minced

1 tablespoon distilled white vinegar

1 tablespoon sugar

1 teaspoon garlic powder

½ teaspoon sea salt

½ teaspoon freshly ground black pepper

In a medium bowl, stir together the yogurt, blue cheese, scallions, vinegar, sugar, garlic powder, salt, and pepper until blended. Refrigerate for 2 hours to let the flavors meld.

STORAGE: Put in an airtight container. Refrigerate for up to 1 week. Freezing is not recommended, because the texture and consistency will change if frozen.

SUBSTITUTION TIP: Replace the plain yogurt with ½ cup mayonnaise and ½ cup sour cream.

Per Serving (1 tablespoon): Calories: 24; Total fat: 1g; Saturated fat: 1g; Protein: 1g; Total carbs: 1g; Fiber: 0g; Sugar: 1g; Sodium: 84mg

Italian Dressing

PREP TIME: 10 MINUTES

This is a versatile dressing. It can be prepared as a vinaigrette or a creamy dressing. The dry seasoning mix can be added to spaghetti sauce, pasta salads, or homemade garlic bread before baking. MAKES 1 CUP

2 tablespoons dried oregano

1½ tablespoons sugar

1 tablespoon onion powder

1 tablespoon garlic powder

1 tablespoon dried parsley

1 teaspoon dried basil

½ teaspoon freshly ground black pepper

½ teaspoon red pepper flakes

¼ teaspoon dried thyme

¼ teaspoon celery seed

¾ cup extra-virgin olive oil

¼ cup balsamic vinegar or distilled white vinegar

1. To make the seasoning mix, in a small bowl, stir together the oregano, sugar, onion powder, garlic powder, parsley, basil, black pepper, red pepper flakes, thyme, and celery seed until blended.

2. In a lidded jar, combine 2 tablespoons of the seasoning mix, the oil, and vinegar. Cover the jar, and shake until combined.

STORAGE: Store the remaining seasoning mix in an airtight container in a cool, dry place for up to 1 year. Refrigerate the prepared dressing in an airtight container for up to 1 week.

VARIATION TIP: For a creamy Italian dressing, in a medium bowl, whisk together 2 tablespoons seasoning mix, 1 cup mayonnaise, ¼ cup diced onion, 2 tablespoons distilled white vinegar, and 1 tablespoon sugar to blend. Put in an airtight container. Refrigerate for up to 5 days.

For a meat marinade, in a medium bowl, whisk together 2 tablespoons dressing mix and 1 cup extra-virgin olive oil until combined. Use to marinate beef, pork, or chicken.

Per Serving (1 tablespoon): Calories: 102; Total fat: 10g; Saturated fat: 1g; Protein: 0g; Total carbs: 3g; Fiber: 0g; Sugar: 2g; Sodium: 2mg

Basic Barbecue Sauce

PREP TIME: 15 MINUTES • COOK TIME: 40 MINUTES

Barbecue sauce recipes vary from state to state and among regions. This Southern-style sauce, with a hint of sweet brown sugar and tangy vinegar, is a wonderful all-purpose sauce for any meat dish. MAKES 3¼ CUPS

2 teaspoons sea salt

1 teaspoon chili powder

1 teaspoon sugar

¾ teaspoon cayenne pepper

½ teaspoon freshly ground
  black pepper

1½ cups tomato sauce

¾ cup distilled white vinegar

½ cup packed light
  brown sugar

½ cup ketchup

2 tablespoons
  prepared mustard

2 tablespoons gluten-free
  Worcestershire sauce

3 tablespoons extra-virgin
  olive oil

3 tablespoons minced garlic

1 white onion, diced

1 bay leaf

1. In a large bowl, whisk together the salt, chili powder, sugar, cayenne, and black pepper until blended.

2. Whisk in the tomato sauce, vinegar, brown sugar, ketchup, mustard, and Worcestershire sauce until smooth.

3. In a large saucepan, combine the oil, garlic, and onion. Cook over medium heat for 5 to 7 minutes, or until the onion is soft and translucent.

4. Stir the tomato sauce mixture into the pan, and add the bay leaf. Bring to a boil, stirring occasionally.

5. Reduce the heat to low. Simmer, stirring occasionally, for 30 minutes, or until the sauce has thickened and reduced by one-fourth. Remove from the heat. Let cool for 20 to 25 minutes.

6. Remove and discard the bay leaf before storing.

STORAGE: Put in an airtight container. Refrigerate for up to 1 week, or freeze for up to 3 months.

THAWING AND REHEATING: Thaw in the refrigerator overnight.

Per Serving (2 tablespoons): Calories: 47; Total Fat: 2g; Saturated Fat: 0g; Protein: 0g; Total Carbs: 8g; Fiber: 1g; Sugar: 6g; Sodium: 255mg

Blueberry Chutney

PREP TIME: 10 MINUTES • COOK TIME: 1 HOUR

This thick, tart blueberry chutney makes for a lovely sandwich spread or can be used as a marinade or topping for chicken or pork, or as the base of a blueberry vinaigrette (see variation tip) for salads. MAKES 2½ CUPS

1 large Granny Smith apple,
  cored and diced
½ cup sugar
½ cup freshly squeezed
  lemon juice
1 teaspoon grated lemon zest
1 teaspoon ground ginger
¼ teaspoon red
  pepper flakes
2 pints fresh blueberries
3 tablespoons
  balsamic vinegar

1. In a medium saucepan, stir together the apple, sugar, lemon juice, lemon zest, ginger, and red pepper flakes. Bring to a boil over medium heat.

2. Reduce the heat to low. Simmer, stirring occasionally, for 15 minutes, or until the mixture has thickened.

3. Stir in the blueberries and vinegar.

4. Increase the heat to high. Bring the chutney to a boil, stirring often.

5. Reduce the heat to low. Cook, stirring occasionally, for 20 minutes, or until the chutney has thickened. Remove from the heat.

STORAGE: Put in an airtight container. Refrigerate for up to 2 weeks, or freeze for up to 3 months.

THAWING AND REHEATING: Thaw in the refrigerator for 4 to 5 hours. Stir before using.

SUBSTITUTION TIP: Use any type of baking apple you like. Jonagold, winesap, or Pink Lady are good choices. Substitute 2 pints blackberries for the blueberries to make blackberry chutney.

VARIATION TIP: For a tangy blueberry vinaigrette, in a medium bowl, whisk together ¼ cup blueberry chutney, ¼ cup minced onion, ⅓ cup balsamic vinegar, 1 teaspoon sea salt, ½ teaspoon freshly ground black pepper, and ⅔ cup canola oil until blended. Put in an airtight container. Refrigerate for up to 2 weeks.

Per Serving (2 tablespoons): Calories: 46; Total fat: 0g; Saturated fat: 0g; Protein: 0g; Total carbs: 12g; Fiber: 1g; Sugar: 9g; Sodium: 1mg

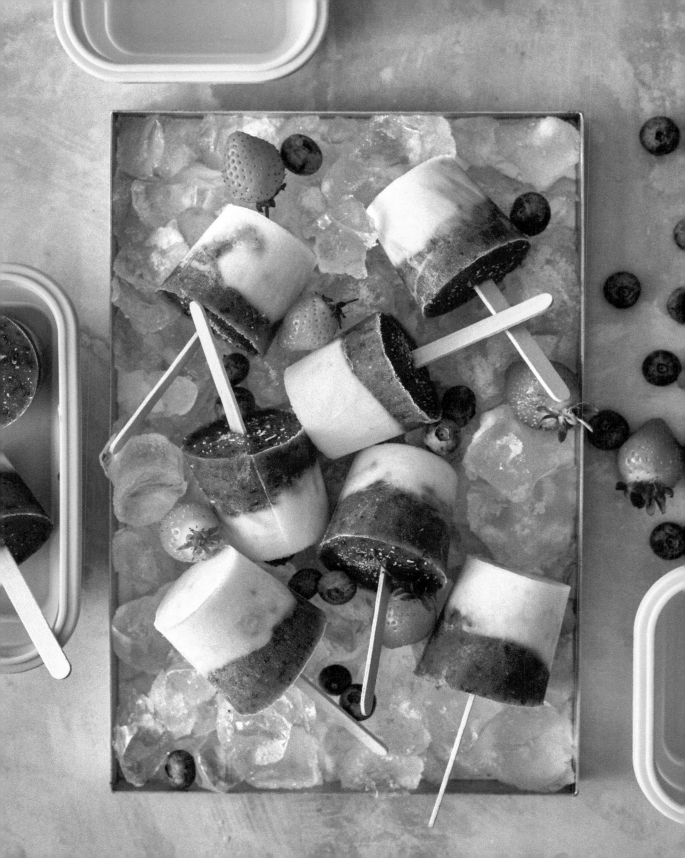

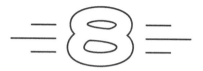

Nibbles and Noshes: Snacks and Desserts

‹‹ Strawberry and Blueberry Yogurt Pops, page 196

Cajun-Spiced Pumpkin Seeds

PREP TIME: 15 MINUTES • COOK TIME: 40 TO 45 MINUTES

Pumpkin seeds are high in fiber, magnesium, and antioxidants. Blended with Cajun seasoning and baked to crunchy perfection, this snack can also be used as a topping for soups and stews. MAKES 1¼ CUPS

Nonstick cooking spray, for coating the sheet pan

1¼ teaspoons paprika

1 teaspoon sea salt

1 teaspoon garlic powder

¾ teaspoon dried thyme

½ teaspoon freshly ground black pepper

½ teaspoon onion powder

½ teaspoon cayenne pepper

½ teaspoon ground cumin

½ teaspoon red pepper flakes

2 (5-ounce) packages raw pumpkin seeds

2 teaspoons extra-virgin olive oil

1. Preheat the oven to 300°F. Line a sheet pan with parchment paper, and coat with cooking spray.

2. In a medium bowl, stir together the paprika, salt, garlic powder, thyme, black pepper, onion powder, cayenne, cumin, and red pepper flakes until blended.

3. Add the pumpkin seeds and oil. Using clean hands, toss the seeds in the seasoning until coated.

4. Evenly spread the pumpkin seeds across the prepared sheet pan.

5. Transfer the sheet pan to the oven, and bake, stirring every 5 to 10 minutes, for 40 to 45 minutes, or until the seeds are golden brown. Remove from the oven. Let cool completely.

STORAGE: Put the cooled seeds in an airtight container. Store at room temperature for up to 2 days, refrigerate for up to 1 week, or freeze for up to 6 months.

THAWING AND REHEATING: Thaw at room temperature for 2 to 3 hours.

SUBSTITUTION TIP: Mixed nuts, peanuts, or sunflower seed kernels can be substituted for the pumpkin seeds.

- -

Per Serving (¼ cup): Calories: 267; Total fat: 13g; Saturated fat: 2g; Protein: 11g; Total carbs: 32g; Fiber: 11g; Sugar: 0g; Sodium: 477mg

Spicy Tortilla Chips

PREP TIME: 10 MINUTES • COOK TIME: 5 TO 10 MINUTES

Did you know you can make crispy tortilla chips at home in less than 20 minutes? These slightly spicy snacks are baked, not fried, but have all the flavor you crave. MAKES 64 CHIPS

1 teaspoon chili powder

¾ teaspoon garlic powder

¾ teaspoon onion powder

½ teaspoon sea salt

2 tablespoons unsalted butter, melted

8 (8-inch) gluten-free flour tortillas

1. Preheat the oven to 400°F.

2. In a small bowl, stir together the chili powder, garlic powder, onion powder, and salt until blended.

3. Stir in the butter.

4. Put the tortillas on a work surface. Evenly spread the butter mixture over the tortillas.

5. Cut each tortilla into 8 wedges, and place the wedges on a sheet pan, leaving room between each wedge.

6. Transfer the sheet pan to the oven, and bake for 6 minutes, or until the wedges are crisp. Remove from the oven. Let cool completely.

STORAGE: Store in an airtight container at room temperature for up to 4 days, or freeze for up to 2 months.

THAWING AND REHEATING: Thaw at room temperature for 30 minutes to 1 hour. The chips can be warmed in the microwave on high power for 30 seconds to give them a freshly baked taste.

SUBSTITUTION TIP: Replace the flour tortillas with corn tortillas or gluten-free pitas.

VARIATION TIP: For cinnamon tortilla chips, in a small bowl, stir together 1 tablespoon sugar and 2 teaspoons ground cinnamon until blended. Omit the spicy seasonings, and prepare as directed.

- -

Per Serving (8 chips): Calories: 178; Total fat: 8g; Saturated fat: 4g; Protein: 3g; Total carbs: 27g; Fiber: 5g; Sugar: 3g; Sodium: 596mg

Olive and Pepper Pinwheels

PREP TIME: 15 MINUTES

An easy, fast, and delicious snack, these bites are packed with a creamy cheese filling and studded with veggies. To make these into sandwich wraps, add 2 or 3 slices of deli turkey or ham to each pinwheel and serve whole. **SERVES 4**

1 (8-ounce) package full-fat cream cheese, at room temperature

½ cup full-fat mayonnaise

½ cup sliced black olives

½ cup shredded sharp Cheddar cheese

2 tablespoons minced scallion, white parts only

2 tablespoons canned diced green chilies

4 (8-inch) gluten-free flour tortillas

1. In a large bowl, combine the cream cheese and mayonnaise. Using a handheld mixer, beat on low speed for 3 to 4 minutes, or until blended.

2. Stir in the olives, Cheddar cheese, scallion, and green chilies.

3. Put the tortillas on a work surface. Evenly spread ½ cup of the cheese mixture over each.

4. Roll the tortillas jelly roll–style, then cut each tortilla into 8 (1-inch-thick) slices.

STORAGE: Put in an airtight container. Refrigerate for up to 5 days, or freeze for up to 2 months.

THAWING AND REHEATING: Thaw in the refrigerator for 4 to 5 hours, or overnight.

INGREDIENT TIP: To keep opened blocks of cream cheese fresh, tightly wrap them in aluminum foil, and store in the coldest part of the refrigerator. Use opened cream cheese within 10 days. Refrigerate unopened cream cheese for up to 1 month. To soften cream cheese, remove it from the wrapper, and put on a microwave-safe dish. Microwave on high power for 15 to 20 seconds.

Per Serving: Calories: 609; Total fat: 82g; Saturated fat: 19g; Protein: 10g; Total carbs: 30g; Fiber: 6g; Sugar: 5g; Sodium: 967mg

Cheddar Cheese Wafers

PREP TIME: 20 MINUTES • COOK TIME: 30 TO 40 MINUTES

Cheddar cheese wafers are a popular Southern dish served for any occasion. The flavor of Cheddar shines in these wafers. A slight pop of heat from the cayenne finishes the bite. **MAKES 20 WAFERS**

Nonstick cooking spray, for coating the sheet pan

1½ cups all-purpose gluten-free one-to-one baking flour

1 teaspoon sea salt

¼ teaspoon cayenne pepper

8 tablespoons (1 stick) unsalted butter, melted

2 cups shredded sharp Cheddar cheese

1. Preheat the oven to 250°F. Coat a sheet pan with cooking spray.

2. In a large bowl, whisk together the flour, salt, and cayenne until blended.

3. Stir in the butter and cheese until a dough forms.

4. Transfer the dough to a piece of wax paper, and roll it to ½-inch thickness. Cut into about 20 (¾-inch) squares.

5. Place the squares on the prepared sheet pan, leaving space between each.

6. Transfer the sheet pan to the oven, and bake for 30 to 40 minutes, or until the wafers are crisp. Remove from the oven.

STORAGE: Place in an airtight container in layers with wax paper or parchment paper between each. Refrigerate for up to 5 days, or freeze for up to 2 months.

THAWING AND REHEATING: Thaw in the refrigerator for 4 to 5 hours.

INGREDIENT TIP: Cheese can become crumbly when frozen. The best way to freeze cheese is to shred or grate it, put it in an airtight freezer-safe bag, and freeze for up to 2 months. It can be used in soups, sauces, omelets, and baked goods directly from the freezer.

Per Serving (4 wafers): Calories: 484; Total fat: 34g; Saturated fat: 20g; Protein: 15g; Total carbs: 29g; Fiber: 1g; Sugar: 0g; Sodium: 759mg

Coconut Pie with Coconut Crust

PREP TIME: 20 MINUTES • COOK TIME: 45 TO 50 MINUTES

A classic Southern recipe, this pie becomes naturally gluten-free with the addition of a coconut crust. Coconut Cream Pie Day is celebrated May 8, but you can enjoy this recipe anytime. SERVES 8

For the crust

Nonstick cooking spray, for coating the pie pan

1½ cups flaked sweetened coconut

3 tablespoons unsalted butter, melted

For the filling

1½ cups sugar

8 tablespoons (1 stick) unsalted butter, melted

3 large eggs, beaten

2 tablespoons freshly squeezed lemon juice

1 teaspoon vanilla extract

1½ cups flaked sweetened coconut

To make the crust

1. Preheat the oven to 325°F. Coat a 9-inch pie pan with cooking spray.

2. In a medium bowl, stir together the coconut and butter until blended.

3. Evenly press the coconut mixture across the bottom and sides of the prepared pie pan.

4. Transfer the pie pan to the oven, and bake for 12 to 15 minutes, or until the coconut turns light brown. Remove from the oven, leaving the oven on.

To make the filling

5. Increase the oven temperature to 350°F.

6. In a medium bowl, combine the sugar and butter. Using a handheld mixer, beat on medium speed for about 3 minutes, or until the mixture is light and fluffy.

7. Turn off the mixer. Stir in the eggs, lemon juice, and vanilla.

8. Add the coconut, and stir until blended.

9. Pour the filling into the piecrust.

10. Return the pie pan to the oven, and bake for 30 to 35 minutes, or until a knife inserted into the center of the pie comes out clean. Remove from the oven.

STORAGE: Put in an airtight container. Refrigerate for up to 3 days, or freeze for up to 3 months.

THAWING AND REHEATING: Thaw in the refrigerator for 6 to 8 hours.

INGREDIENT TIP: A package of unopened flaked coconut can be stored in the pantry for 6 months, or frozen for 6 to 8 months. Thaw at room temperature for 1 hour before using.

Per Serving: Calories: 489; Total fat: 30g; Saturated fat: 22g; Protein: 4g; Total carbs: 55g; Fiber: 2g; Sugar: 53g; Sodium: 121mg

Chocolate Brownie Pie

PREP TIME: 15 MINUTES • COOK TIME: 20 TO 25 MINUTES

Rich, fudgy, dark chocolate. Sprinkles of pecans. This pie is loaded with both, making it a dessert for any occasion. Add a dollop of whipped cream to push it over the top. SERVES 8

Nonstick cooking spray, for coating the baking dish

2 (1-ounce) squares unsweetened baking chocolate, melted

8 tablespoons (1 stick) salted butter, melted

1 cup sugar

2 large eggs, beaten

½ cup pecans, chopped

Whipped cream, for serving (optional)

1. Preheat the oven to 350°F. Coat a 9-by-9-inch baking dish with cooking spray.

2. In a large bowl, combine the chocolate and butter. Using a handheld mixer, blend on medium speed for 3 to 4 minutes, or until smooth.

3. To make the batter, add the sugar and eggs. Mix for about 3 minutes, or until creamy.

4. Turn off the mixer. Stir in the pecans.

5. Pour the batter into the prepared baking dish, and cover with aluminum foil.

6. Transfer the baking dish to the oven, and bake for 20 minutes.

7. Remove the foil, and bake for 5 more minutes, if needed, or until a knife inserted into the center comes out clean. Remove from the oven. Let cool for 20 minutes.

8. Serve the pie with whipped cream (if using).

STORAGE: Tightly wrap the pie in foil, and put it in an airtight container. Store at room temperature for up to 2 days, refrigerate for up to 4 days, or freeze for up to 3 months.

THAWING AND REHEATING: Thaw at room temperature for 1 to 2 hours. Individual thawed slices of pie can be put on a microwave-safe plate and heated in the microwave on high power for 5 to 10 seconds.

Per Serving: Calories: 309; Total fat: 21g; Saturated fat: 10g; Protein: 3g; Total carbs: 28g; Fiber: 2g; Sugar: 25g; Sodium: 21mg

Triple-Berry Parfaits

PREP TIME: 20 MINUTES

"Parfait" means "perfect" in French, and these layered fruity snacks fit the bill. Parfaits were first developed in 1894. Our updated version has the flavor of three tart, juicy berries. The parfaits pair perfectly with crunchy homemade granola (see tip), or you can replace the granola with 1 cup toasted chopped almonds, pecans, or walnuts; mini chocolate chips; or raisins, as you like. **SERVES 4**

**1½ cups fresh
   strawberries, hulled**
½ cup fresh blueberries
½ cup fresh raspberries
⅓ cup sugar
3 cups full-fat vanilla yogurt
1 cup gluten-free granola

1. In a food processor or blender, combine the strawberries, blueberries, raspberries, and sugar. Process for 5 to 10 seconds, or until finely chopped.

2. In each of 4 (8-ounce) Mason jars, layer ½ cup of yogurt, and place 2 tablespoons of chopped berries on top. Top the berries with ¼ cup of yogurt, and layer on another 2 tablespoons of chopped berries. Seal the jars.

STORAGE: Refrigerate for up to 3 days, or freeze for up to 3 months. Store the granola in an airtight container at room temperature for up to 1 month, or freeze for up to 3 months.

THAWING AND REHEATING: Thaw in the refrigerator overnight. Add ¼ cup granola to each parfait immediately before serving.

INGREDIENT TIP: Make your own gluten-free granola. Preheat the oven to 200°F. Line a sheet pan with parchment paper, and coat with cooking spray. In a large bowl, stir together 3 cups gluten-free old-fashioned rolled oats, ½ cup honey, ½ cup canola oil, and 1 teaspoon sea salt. Evenly spread the granola across the prepared sheet pan. Bake for 20 minutes, stirring halfway through. Remove from the oven. Let cool, and break into pieces. Store in an airtight container for up to 1 week, or freeze for up to 3 months.

Per Serving: Calories: 363; Total fat: 13g; Saturated fat: 9g; Protein: 10g; Total carbs: 51g; Fiber: 5g; Sugar: 35g; Sodium: 176mg

Strawberry and Blueberry Yogurt Pops

PREP TIME: 15 MINUTES

Yogurt pops provide a cool, refreshing snack on hot days. Loaded with fresh fruit, these creamy treats can be made in minutes. Adjust the sugar for personal preference, or replace the water with fruit juice. MAKES 10 POPS

¾ **cup fresh blueberries**

¾ **cup fresh strawberries, hulled**

¼ **cup sugar**

¼ **cup water**

2½ **cups full-fat key lime yogurt**

1. In a blender or food processor, combine the blueberries, strawberries, sugar, and water. Blend for 10 seconds, or until pureed.

2. Line up 10 (3-ounce) paper cups, and pour ¼ cup yogurt into each cup.

3. Spoon 2 tablespoons of the pureed fruit into each cup over the yogurt.

4. Place an ice pop stick into each cup, and stir to blend.

5. Cover each cup with aluminum foil, and freeze for 2 to 3 hours, or until firm.

STORAGE: Remove the yogurt pops from the paper cups, and put the pops in an airtight freezer-safe container. Freeze for up to 3 months.

SUBSTITUTION TIP: Use your favorite flavor of fruit yogurt and berries. Good combinations include raspberry and banana with raspberry yogurt, or peach and mango with peach yogurt.

Per Serving (1 yogurt pop): Calories: 67; Total fat: 2g; Saturated fat: 1g; Protein: 2g; Total carbs: 10g; Fiber: 1g; Sugar: 9g; Sodium: 28mg

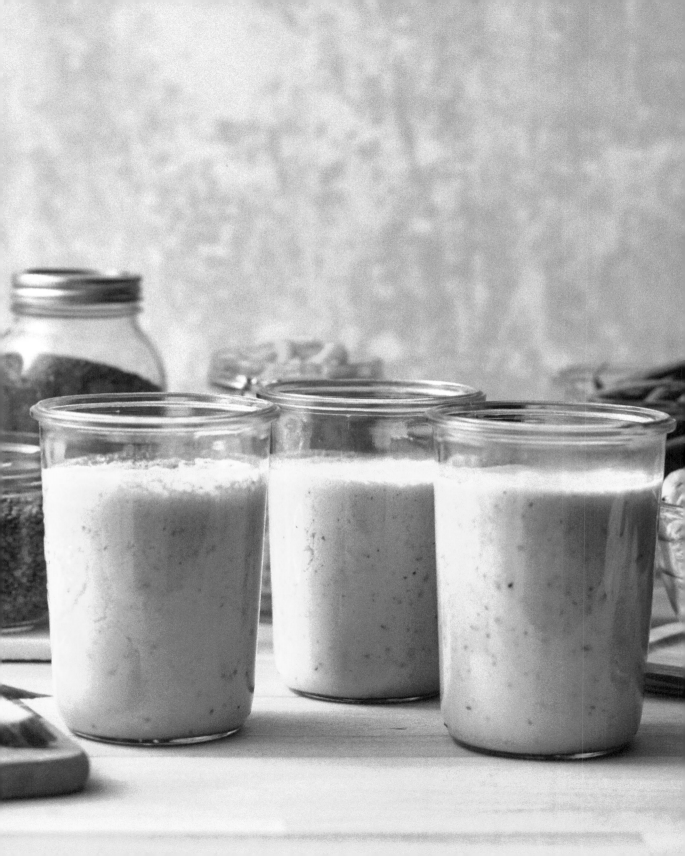

Measurement Conversions

Volume Equivalents (Liquid)

US STANDARD	US STANDARD (OUNCES)	METRIC (APPROXIMATE)
2 tablespoons	1 fl. oz.	30 mL
¼ cup	2 fl. oz.	60 mL
½ cup	4 fl. oz.	120 mL
1 cup	8 fl. oz.	240 mL
1½ cups	12 fl. oz.	355 mL
2 cups or 1 pint	16 fl. oz.	475 mL
4 cups or 1 quart	32 fl. oz.	1 L
1 gallon	128 fl. oz.	4 L

Oven Temperatures

FAHRENHEIT (F)	CELSIUS (C) (APPROXIMATE)
250°F	120°C
300°F	150°C
325°F	165°C
350°F	180°C
375°F	190°C
400°F	200°C
425°F	220°C
450°F	230°C

Volume Equivalents (Dry)

US STANDARD	METRIC (APPROXIMATE)
⅛ teaspoon	0.5 mL
¼ teaspoon	1 mL
½ teaspoon	2 mL
¾ teaspoon	4 mL
1 teaspoon	5 mL
1 tablespoon	15 mL
¼ cup	59 mL
⅓ cup	79 mL
½ cup	118 mL
⅔ cup	156 mL
¾ cup	177 mL
1 cup	235 mL
2 cups or 1 pint	475 mL
3 cups	700 mL
4 cups or 1 quart	1 L

Weight Equivalents

US STANDARD	METRIC (APPROXIMATE)
½ ounce	15 g
1 ounce	30 g
2 ounces	60 g
4 ounces	115 g
8 ounces	225 g
12 ounces	340 g
16 ounces or 1 pound	455 g

References

Gill, Chuck. "Study Suggests U.S. Households Waste Nearly a Third of the Food They Acquire." *Penn State News*, September 2, 2020. News.psu .edu/story/602482/2020/01/23/research/study-suggests-us-households -waste-nearly-third-food-they-acquire

United States Department of Agriculture. "Food Prices and Spending." Economic Research Service. Last modified July 17, 2020. ERS.usda .gov/data-products/ag-and-food-statistics-charting-the-essentials /food-prices-and-spending

Index

Acknowledgments

Thanks to my publisher, Rockridge Press/Callisto Media, Inc., for the chance to try a new cookbook genre. Thanks to the editorial staff; Susan Haynes, for thinking of me when thinking of gluten-free; Myryah Irby, for her patience, encouragement, and guidance; and to the production team. Thanks, also, to Mike Deweese for the lovely author photo.

I'd like to thank my family: my husband, Bryan, and my son, Ashton, for taste-testing the recipes and offering critiques and for grilling hamburgers when I was too busy to cook; my daughter, Brittany, son-in-law, Justin, and granddaughter, "Critter," for sampling everything in my refrigerator to "make sure it tastes good;" my friend, Dawn McAlexander, for her support and advice; and all of my family, friends, and readers who have encouraged me through comments, emails, and messages.

About the Author

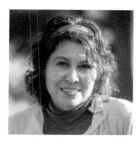 **Pam Wattenbarger** began experimenting with recipe creation as a teen and hasn't looked back. When her daughter was diagnosed with celiac disease in 2010, she turned her efforts toward preparing gluten-free goodies she is proud to share with family and friends. If she's not baking or cooking, you can find her daydreaming of travel or browsing through her vast selection of cookbooks. Connect with Pam at her website, SimplySouthernMom.com, or in her Facebook group, Simply Southern Recipes & Tips.

CPSIA information can be obtained
at www.ICGtesting.com
Printed in the USA
BVHW020953181120
593622BV00017B/410